ANIMAL SENSES

ANIMAL SENSES

Robert Burton

DAVID & CHARLES : NEWTON ABBOT

Reprinted in 1973

Printed in Great Britain
by Redwood Press Ltd Trowbridge Wiltshire
for David & Charles (Holdings) Ltd
South Devon House Newton Abbot Devon

Contents

Illustrations

PLATES

DIAGRAMS IN THE TEXT

8

CHAPTER ONE

Understanding animals

We live in a world bounded by the limits of our senses and for
centuries we have assumed that this is the only world. Then, as
the explorers and scientists of the fifteenth and sixteenth centuries showed that the boundaries of the world, and the universe, stretched far beyond anything previously imagined, so
biologists of the twentieth century have shown that there are
sensory worlds outside our own that are often hardly be-
lievable in extent. We know now that there are sounds beyond
the range of our hearing; that we cannot perceive them does not
mean that they do not exist. Similarly we know that there are
smells and sights that are beyond us and that there are senses
that we do not possess.

Anyone who has kept pets knows that animals often have
keener senses than human beings. Dogs can smell odours in-
finitely weaker than any of which we are conscious and cats see
their way in light conditions that we would term 'pitch dark'. In
these instances the animals are using senses little different from
ours, except that their sense organs are more sensitive. Their
world is just that bit brighter than ours, and it is also larger in
some respects. The boundaries have been pushed back, for their
sense organs are receptive to sights, sounds or smells beyond our
capacity. Our ears can detect sounds up to 20,000 cps, but dogs
can hear frequencies of up to 40,000 cps and can be trained to
respond to a Galton 'silent' whistle. Blowing a Galton whistle
produces a sound too high for us to hear, but a dog will react
instantly.

These differences are only a matter of degree, but there also

9

exist senses quite beyond human imagination which add new dimensions to a world that, for us, is limited by our traditional five senses. How can we fully appreciate that some kinds of fish or termites are sensitive to magnetic fields, for example, when barriers exist even between one human being and another? A colour-blind person is unable to appreciate painting, those who are tone-deaf cannot enjoy music, and how can a person with normal senses explain colours and tunes to such people? The idea that some people may be living in a narrower world has brought a more sympathetic appreciation of their difficulties; the backward child may not be mentally deficient, but merely suffering from some defect in sight or hearing that robs him of information about his surroundings.

If it is so difficult for us to get inside the minds of others of our own kind, to see things as they see them, how much more difficult it is to see the world through the senses of a fly, a bat or a skate; yet unless we can understand the kind of world an animal lives in, studies of its behaviour have very little meaning. The following chapters examine how animals make use of their senses in different ways to regulate their lives: to find food, mates and shelter, or to escape from enemies. We shall see how their sense organs are used to collect the necessary information. In other words, we will see the different worlds that animals live in or, more precisely, how they react to their different environments. An animal's environment is the sum total of the external influences that act on it and it is these influences that its sense organs have to register.

Before exploring some of the different worlds that animals live in, the part that sense organs play in their lives must be explained and an account of the ways scientists study senses must be given. At the simplest level, an animal's behaviour can be represented by the diagram on the following page.

The sense organ receives information or stimuli from the environment in the form of energy such as light or sound waves. The information is then coded and relayed by the nerves to the brain or central nervous system. The latter term is usually pre-

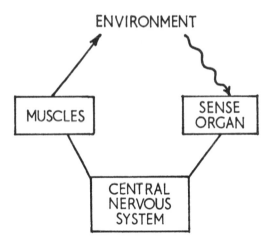

ferred by scientists because many simple animals do not have any special concentration of nerve cells that could be called a brain, and even in advanced animals some information is dealt with in the spinal cord, without ever being passed through the brain.

In the central nervous system the information is sorted and correlated with information from other sense organs or from the memory. A decision is then made as to what action the animal is to take in response to what it has learnt about its environment. For the decision to be implemented, impulses are sent by the nerves to the muscles. The whole effect of this sequence is for the animal to modify its environment, or more often for the animal to move to a new and more favourable environment. Thus a woodlouse moves from a dry to a moist environment under a log or stone and a mouse released on a lawn scuttles to the shelter of a hedge. On receiving adverse stimuli both have moved position so that their environment no longer contains those stimuli. The interaction of environment and an animal's senses can be seen as a continually regulating system designed to bring the greatest benefit to the animal. This is an important point to consider during the following pages. Two parts of this system, the sense organs and behaviour, are our concern here. The workings of the sense organs are considered in detail, but the mechanism of the central nervous system, in so far as it is known, and the muscle systems are beyond the scope of this book. Instead, the behaviour of an animal as a whole is described in relation to the sense organs.

Sense organs have a basic structure and mechanism, expressed thus:

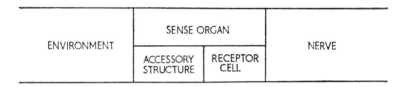

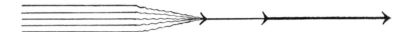

Each sense organ receives energy in one form or another from the environment. There are two basic types of sense organs: contact receptors and distance receptors. The former includes the organs of taste and touch which receive stimuli from objects in contact with the animal's body. Distance receptors such as eyes, ears and nose gather information which may have been weakened by travelling over some distance and so need collecting and modifying by the sense organ. The information is transformed in the sense organ into a series of nerve impulses. This is known as transduction; a microphone, for instance, is a transducer that converts sound energy into electrical energy. A carbon disc in the microphone head bends under the minute pressure of sound waves. As it bends, its electrical resistance decreases allowing an electric current to flow through it more strongly. Biological transducers, the receptor cells in sense organs, transduce energy from the environment into electric energy in much the same way. Stimulation of the receptor cell sets up an electric current, the receptor potential. This spreads to the nerve fibre and triggers a powerful nerve impulse.

A large proportion of our knowledge of biological trans-duction has been gained from studies of a simple receptor cell called the Pacinian corpuscle, which is sensitive to pressure, or bending. Pacinian corpuscles are found in many parts of the body, in the skin, muscles and joints. We are not conscious of their working but they are continually measuring the stresses and strains on different parts of our bodies. They are parti-cularly useful for experiments because they are large and can be easily separated from the surrounding tissue. A good place to find them is in the mesentery, the very fine, transparent mem-brane that suspends the intestine from the wall of the abdomen. Pacinian corpuscles, together with their connecting nerve fibres, can be cut from the mesentery and kept alive for several hours, responding to pressure as they would in the body.

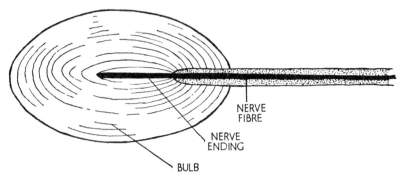

Fig 1   Pacinian corpuscle with the bare nerve ending surrounded by a bulb of fine layers of tissue. Pressure on the bulb bends the nerve ending firing nerve impulses along the nerve fibre

A Pacinian corpuscle is onion-shaped, 1 mm long and $\frac{1}{2}$ mm thick. The fine ending of the nerve fibre is surrounded by layers of tissue forming a bulb like an onion. When a minute pressure is exerted on the bulb, bending it slightly, a series of nerve impulses is set off. If all the layers of the bulb are then stripped away, nerve impulses can still be recorded, which means that the site of the transducer must be in the nerve ending in the centre of the bulb. By carefully altering the degree of bending and recording the subsequent nerve impulses, it has been found that the more the Pacinian corpuscle is bent, the greater is the frequency of the nerve impulses. So the central nervous system is informed about the stresses and strains in the body by a simple code, in which the extent to which the receptor cell bends is signalled by the number of nerve impulses arriving each second.

A long series of experiments has solved some of the mysteries of the way in which pressure on the Pacinian corpuscle is changed into nerve impulses. We have a fairly clear picture of what the process of transduction is even if we do not fully understand how it works. There is a close analogy between the sense cell and the microphone. In the Pacinian corpuscle, as in other receptor cells, there is a continuous electric charge in the nerve ending which changes as the membrane surrounding it is distorted.

The continuous charge in the sense cell is caused by the difference in the concentration of ions (charged atoms or molecules) on either side of the membrane. There is a higher concentration of positive ions on the exterior so that the outside of the cell is positively charged with respect to the inside. When the cell membrane is distorted it somehow 'springs a leak' and the positive ions flood in, reversing the electric charge. Quite how light, heat, chemical, pressure or other forms of energy effect this is not known, but the result is that the altered charge, the receptor potential, spreads over the surface of the receptor cell and, if it is strong enough, triggers an explosive impulse in the connecting nerve fibre. Afterwards the cell membrane is re-sealed and the original difference in ion concentration built up.

Before any part of this sequence can happen, energy from the environment has to reach the receptor cell. On the way, it is modified by accessory structures, such as the lens and pupil of the eye. Some energy is filtered out, so that right from the start the animal is selecting information from the bewildering array that is bombarding it. In bright light, for instance, the pupil contracts so that the amount of light entering the eye is cut down and it is not blinded, and the lens concentrates light on the receptor cells of the retina so that the information they pass on is more detailed.

Another important function of the filtering mechanism is to select the kind of energy to be passed on as the receptor cells are not sensitive to only one particular kind of energy. The lens and other structures of the eye allow only light to stimulate the receptor cells in the retina, as the brain is designed to accept only visual information from the eyes. A simple way of 'fooling' the brain is to press the eyes with the fingers. The pressure stimulates the receptor cells in the retina and the brain interprets this pressure as light and we see brilliant flashes. Scientists have also been fooled by the sensitivity of sense cells to different kinds of energy. Skates and rays, belonging to the group known as 'cartilaginous fishes', because their skeletons are made of soft cartilage rather than hard bone, have sense organs called the ampullae of Lorenzini, so named after the man who discovered them. These organs lie in pits in the skin and careful experiments showed that they reacted to pressure and to temperature. As pressure receptors they would be able to detect pressure waves in the water, but there seemed no apparent reason for having temperature receptors lying so deep in the skin. Eventually, they were found to have a quite different function. They are extremely sensitive to electric currents and, by comparison, relatively insensitive to pressure or temperature, which are just side effects like the flashing lights caused by pressure on the eyeballs. The function of the ampullae of Lorenzini and other electric-sensitive organs is discussed in more detail in Chapter Eleven.

The differences between the sense organs of lowly animals, such as earthworms or sea anemones, and those of mammals or birds lie mainly in the complexity of the accessory structures. The well-developed, complex structures in the eyes, ears and other organs of higher animals increase the sensitivity of the organs because they cut down or narrow the range of energy entering them, so that while each organ is taking note of only a small part of the total environment, this small part is studied intensively. With knowledge of the fine details, the animal's behaviour can be much more sophisticated. An earthworm with simple light-sensitive organs can do no more than tell the difference between strong and weak light and its only response to light is to move towards or away from the light source. Compare this with man who can see a three-dimensional, moving, coloured world of images and who can adapt his behaviour in response to a single image or a pattern of many.

As a first step in studying animal senses one can make a rough guess as to which senses an animal uses most merely by watching it. A cat has large eyes with pupils that dilate at night so it is reasonable to suppose that it can see well in dim light. A mole, on the other hand, has eyes like pinheads so we assume that it uses some other sense to find out about its environment. The next step is to watch an animal under set conditions, altering its environment to see how it reacts, so obtaining an idea of its behaviour in relation to its environment. Tests like these gave the first information about the behaviour of simple animals and laid the foundations for the study of the more complex behaviour of advanced animals.

It is not difficult to see how simple animals react to features of their environment: a lighted window attracts moths and food left lying about attracts flies (although this tells very little about the nature of the attraction). Quite simple tests will show how simple animals react, because they have very poorly developed central nervous systems and their behaviour is simple and rigid. Give such an animal a stimulus in the form of some sort of energy from its environment and it will react in a standard way which will be repeated time after time. Yet simple as it is, this behaviour is sufficient for the needs of the animal. It leads it to the most favourable conditions of temperature and humidity, enables it to find food and brings the sexes together for breeding.

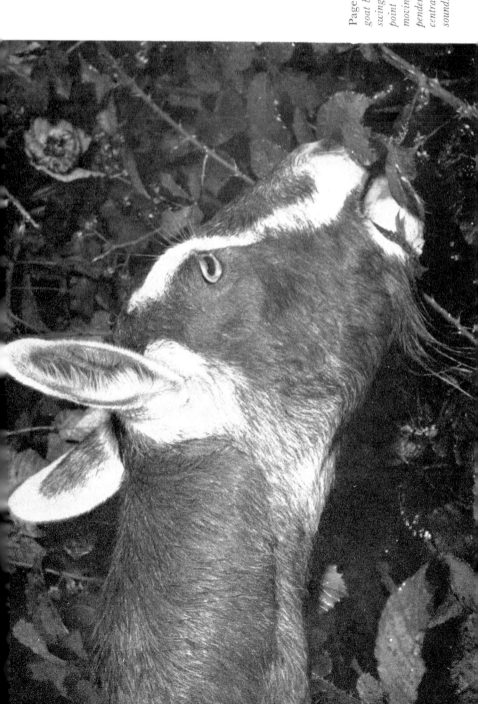

Page 17 *As this goat browses, its ears swing round to pinpoint sounds. By moving them independently it can concentrate on two sounds at once*

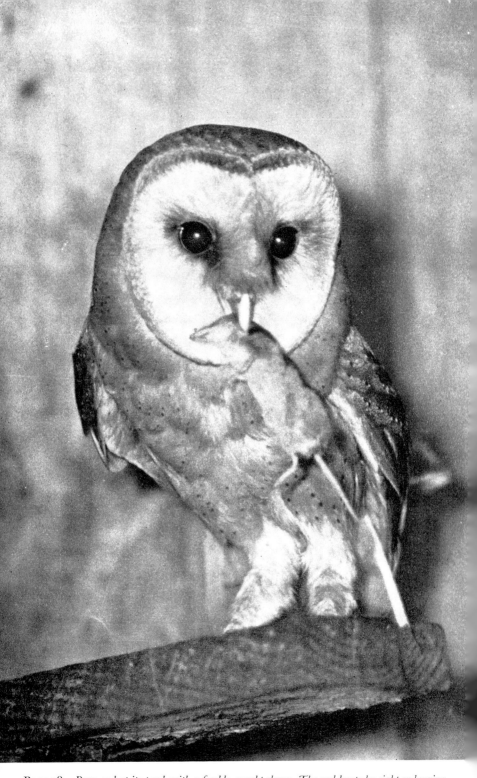

Barn owl at its perch with a freshly-caught shrew. The owl hunts by sight or hearing, both incredibly keen. The shrew's only defence is to keep hidden

Among the simpler animals, woodlice belong to the large group of arthropods, or joint-legged animals. This group includes insects, spiders, scorpions, shrimps, crabs, water fleas and many others. The nearest relatives to woodlice are the shrimps, crabs and water fleas, and they all belong to the subdivision of arthropods called crustaceans. Most crustaceans live in water but some, like the woodlouse, live on land, and unlike other land-living arthropods, the insects, spiders and scorpions, the hard outer skin of the woodlouse is not watertight. If kept in a dry place a woodlouse soon dries up and dies. It is not surprising, therefore, that woodlice seek damp places to live, and are usually found under stones, or under the loose bark of dead trees.

The moisture-seeking behaviour of woodlice can be easily demonstrated with simple apparatus. A dish can be divided into wet and dry halves by placing shallow trays in it, one containing water-absorbing sulphuric acid and the other water. A gauze floor is placed over the trays and woodlice allowed to run around in the arena so formed. In a short time they will settle down on the moist side of the dish. The mechanism with which they respond is called a kinesis, in which an animal reacts to a stimulus by moving around. It wanders about at random until the stimulus ends, whereupon the animal stops moving. This is how the woodlice behave. They are sensitive to the humidity of the air about them: when it is dry they move about; when it is moist they stop, and in this way woodlice finish up in the moist half of the dish, or, in their natural environment, under stones and bark.

In a more complex form of kinesis, an animal moves in a straight line when in favourable conditions but as soon as it enters conditions less favourable, it starts moving in circles. If the circling brings it back into more favourable conditions again, it straightens its course. Insects react in this way, but the process seems to be a haphazard one for the insect cannot tell from which direction the favourable stimulus is coming. There seems to be no sense of purpose about this behaviour as there is, for instance, in a moth flying into a candle. (It is, obviously, incorrect to talk about purpose in describing such a mechanical piece of behaviour, as this implies that the moth is thinking about what it is doing, but to anyone comparing the two animals it describes the difference observed between the meandering of the woodlouse and the direct flight of the moth.)

The moth's behaviour as it flies towards a light is called a taxis, a form of simple behaviour in which the animal's reactions are directed by a more complex system of sense organs. In taxic behaviour the animal steers itself by comparing the strength of the stimuli on either side of its body. It can do this indirectly by turning continually from side to side or directly by comparing the stimuli simultaneously by paired sense organs, such as eyes or ears that are placed one on each side of the head. If the stimulus is favourable, the animal turns towards the side that is more strongly stimulated until it is facing the source of the stimulus. This evens the stimulus on either side and the animal moves straight towards the source. If the stimulus is unfavourable, the animal turns away from it.

A more detailed way of finding out the sensitivity of sense organs is to carry out experiments on conditioned reflexes, which constitute a simple form of learning. This is a technique made famous by Pavlov's experiments on dogs, whilst he was studying the mechanism controlling the secretion of digestive juices. When meat is placed in a dog's mouth, it automatically salivates, the saliva being used to lubricate food in the mouth so that it can be swallowed easily: it is a complete reflex action, over which there is no control. Pavlov, however, found that the dogs soon started to salivate before they received the food, having learnt to recognise the various actions that preceded the meal. He then trained his dogs to salivate to order by ringing a bell before feeding them, and after a while the dogs would salivate at the sound of a bell, even if they were given no food. This is the essence of a conditioned reflex, to which humans are just as prone as dogs: a simple reflex (food in mouth → salivation) is triggered by an unusual stimulus (sound of bell, smell or sight of food) because of its associations. There is no need for the associations to be fulfilled.

For this reason, conditioned reflexes are of great use in studying the capacities of sense organs. An animal can be trained to respond to all manner of stimuli that are not connected with the original piece of reflex behaviour. If, for example, a dog is trained to associate a whistle with food, it is possible to find out how high a pitch the dog can hear by adjusting a Galton whistle to produce higher and higher pitched notes. The dog would fail to salivate as soon as the pitch became too high for it to hear.

The simplest conditioned reflex experiment can be done with an earthworm which can be made to crawl down a tube ending in a T-junction. If it is given an electric shock every time it turns right, the worm eventually learns to turn left, and will continue to turn left each time it reaches the T-junction. From this experiment we learn that earthworms can tell left from right, but more complex experiments can give very much more detailed information on an animal's capabilities. In Chapter Six experiments on the colour vision of honeybees are described. By a long series of experiments conditioning bees to associate a particular colour with the presence of food, it was possible to find out precisely which colours bees are able to distinguish.

Until about twenty years ago our knowledge of the workings of sense organs was based mainly on experiments using conditioned reflexes, but there are drawbacks. The method is extremely time consuming. To find out the highest note dogs can hear it is necessary to test a variety of dogs and to test each one several times, and even then it is not possible to be certain that the correct deduction has been made. Guinea pigs were thought to have poor hearing as it was difficult to condition them to noises. It is now known that guinea pigs can hear quite well but that their reaction to sound is to keep still, and this is why they seemed to make no response to the test noises. This is a fault in the method which has to be watched continually. The animal's senses may respond to the energy from a certain stimulus but that does not mean that the animal's behaviour will show that it has received the stimulus. Now, however, methods have been developed for listening in directly to the messages running up the nerves from the sense organs.

The technique of tapping nerve fibres was invented about forty years ago. The method was the same as that of tapping telephone cables. One electrode was merely stuck into the body, earthed so to speak, while the other was connected to a nerve fibre. The tapped current could be amplified in a loudspeaker so that each impulse was heard as a click, or could be seen as a trace on an oscilloscope. Once the electrodes were in place the sense organ could be tested with a whole range of stimuli in a comparatively short time, but here again there was a limitation. The messages passing down the nerve were from the sense organ as a whole, because a single nerve is made up of hundreds of fibres each carrying its own messages. It was only possible to study individual sense cells when they could be found in isolation, as with the Pacinian corpuscle. Later extremely fine microelectrodes were made so that messages passing up individual nerve fibres could be recorded. It has even been possible, by placing microelectrodes within the cells, to detect the electric charge spreading across the membrane of a receptor cell to trigger the nerve impulse.

Together with study by microelectrodes, sense organs are being investigated by electron microscopy. Extremely thin sections of tissue are photographed with a stream of electrons instead of the light which is utilised in an ordinary microscope. The very high magnifications that can be obtained show incredibly minute structures within the sense and nerve cells and these can be related to the electrical changes revealed by the use of microelectrodes. Microelectrodes and the electron microscope have revolutionised studies of sense organs and sense cells. Their use has, for example, invalidated the previously accepted theory of the mechanism of the compound eyes of insects (Chapter Six). Every year sees new advances and scientific journals are so full of new information that it is difficult to digest it all. Indeed there is a danger of not being able to see the wood for the trees.

It is possible for a wealth of data to be collected on the working of various parts of a sense organ without anyone being much the wiser as to its overall function. What is worse, studies of sense organ function are becoming divorced from natural conditions. Instead of working on a whole animal, a small piece of it is used. Its reactions are not being related to its environment but to a light source or an artificially produced noise of pure tone. By tapping the sense organs near their source we are learning about the responses of a sense organ, not the perceptions of an animal. At one time, for instance, the eyes of the king crab were known to be sensitive to light but no one had shown that the animal actually responded to light or that light modified its behaviour.

The biologists who do this work are well aware of these shortcomings and of the necessity of supplementing their microscopic techniques with studies on animal behaviour. The studies on sense organs and the important ideas as to their function, which are emerging from the laboratory, should not be slighted but the animals must be followed into the countryside. For an animal does not see a light source, it sees the surrounding scenery from which it has to select the important images to determine its behaviour. Carefully watching animals in their natural surroundings and relating their behaviour to laboratory studies of their sense organs will show us what use animals really make of their senses, what sort of a world they live in and why they behave as they do.

Some of these findings are presented in the following chapters. No attempt is made to include all the senses, and after a description of the mechanism of a sense organ only a few examples of its use are given to show in detail how animals use different information from their environment to perform various tasks: finding their homes and their food or escaping from enemies. Very often they are using information that is outside the bounds of our world and can only be detected by sophisticated instruments. This makes study more difficult but more interesting as it unlocks secrets of nature that we did not know existed even a few years ago.

CHAPTER TWO

Listening for trouble

Before describing the mechanism of the ear it is necessary to get a clear idea of what sound is. It is a movement of energy through a medium, but the medium itself does not move; sound can travel through a solid medium, such as a brick wall, and the particles of brick do not travel from one side of the wall to the other, but they do oscillate as the sound energy passes.

A tuning fork or the string of a guitar oscillates when plucked. The vibration of the string imparts vibration to the surrounding particles of air which spread the motion to their neighbours so that there is an alternating series of compressions and decom-

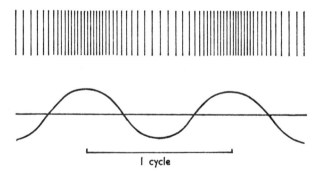

I cycle

Fig 2   Representation of sound waves moving across the page. Sound waves consist of alternate compression and rarefaction of the medium, although the particles of the medium do not move bodily with the sound. Underneath is the conventional representation of sound waves, indicating 1 cycle. The frequency of a sound is expressed as the number of cycles that pass a point in 1 sec. The distance between the top and bottom of crests is the amplitude of the sound and is a measure of the loudness

pressions, with the air pressure rising and falling. This movement of particles is represented graphically by a series of waves. The peaks of the waves represent the compressions and the troughs between them the decompressions. The speed at which the waves pass through the medium is the speed of the sound. In air, sound travels at 750 mph at sea level and aeroplanes that fly faster than this are said to break the sound barrier. At high altitudes where the air is thin, the speed of sound drops and planes break the sound barrier at a speed considerably less than the 750 mph of sea level. Conversely, sound travels faster through a denser medium like water and faster still through rock.

The number of waves that pass a point each second is an expression of the 'frequency' of the sound. Each peak and trough represents one cycle, and sound frequency or pitch is expressed as cycles per second or cps. A sound of high pitch has a high frequency, while a low-pitched sound has a low frequency. The distance between two peaks or two troughs is called the wavelength. It is easy to see that if the wavelength is decreased, the frequency, or the number of waves per second, will be increased.

The human ear, or the ear of any other animal, is sensitive to only a restricted range of frequencies or wavelengths. Pressure waves below 20 cps are not registered by our ears as sounds, but are felt as vibrations through our bodies. At the other end of the scale, we cannot hear vibrations above about 20,000 cps. Frequencies above this are termed 'ultrasonic', that is, beyond sound. There is no special property of these sounds, it is just a convenient name for sounds too high for humans to hear. Some animals can hear sounds well above 20,000 cps and the importance of ultrasonic hearing is discussed in Chapter Four.

The upper limit of hearing varies from person to person and, in general, children can hear sounds of higher pitch than adults. This is very nicely illustrated by the story of a small boy, aged four, who woke his parents one night, making a great fuss. As he was rarely any trouble at night, both parents went to his room. He complained that something had been flying around the room, squeaking. The parents could see nothing and tried to quieten him, but the boy became more upset, insisting desperately that something had definitely been there. Eventually he cried out that it had started to squeak again and to reassure him, his parents started to search every corner of the room. In due course they found a bat clinging to one of the curtains. The boy could hear its squeaks but his parents could not.

Now, it must be emphasised that these squeaks were not the same as the ultrasonic impulses used for echo-location that are described in Chapter Four. They were the same as the squeaks made by mice communicating with other mice. The importance of the story is that it illustrates that it cannot even be taken for granted that one human appreciates the same sounds, or sights and smells, as another. And when studying other animals, one

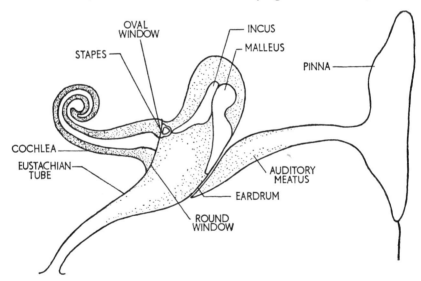

Fig 3 Diagrammatic representation of the human ear. Sound is collected by the pinna and transmitted down the auditory meatus to the eardrum where it is carried by the three ear bones, the malleus, incus and stapes to the round window of the cochlea. In the cochlea sound waves are converted into nerve impulses. The eustachian leads from the mouth and equalises air pressure on either side of the eardrum. The semicircular canals, concerned with balance and movement, have been omitted for clarity

must work from the premise that their range of experience may be totally different.

Another characteristic of sound waves is the intensity or loudness of the sound which is represented by the distance of the peak or the trough from the mid-line. This is also a measure of the energy of that sound.

Sound waves set up by the vibration of a guitar string, tuning fork or other source are collected by the external ear or pinna and travel down the auditory meatus, whose only translation into everyday English is the unlovely 'ear-hole', to the eardrum. This is a membrane, 1 cm in diameter, that vibrates as the sound waves hit it, so forming the first stage of the transducer. The vibrations are amplified and passed on to the receptor cells of the inner ear by the mechanism of the middle ear.

The middle ear is a chamber, called the bulla, containing three small bones, or ossicles, that hinge one against the other. Their names are the malleus, incus and stapes, or hammer, anvil and stirrup. The base of the malleus rests against the eardrum and vibrates as the eardrum vibrates. The vibration is transmitted from the malleus, through the incus to the stirrup-shaped stapes that rests in the opening of the oval window, leading to the inner ear. The oval window is eighteen times smaller than the eardrum so that the ossicles of the middle ear are acting as an amplifier, magnifying pressure exerted on the eardrum about eighteen times.

To prevent the inner ear being damaged by the amplification of too loud a sound, special muscles attached to the malleus and the stapes can contract, drawing the malleus and stapes away from the eardrum and the oval window. Sound can still pass through but its intensity is very much reduced.

The inner ear consists of two fluid-filled structures embedded in the bone of the skull. The semicircular canals are organs of balance and they may be left out of a discussion on hearing. Lying under them is the cochlea, consisting of a spiral tube like the shell of a snail. The cochlea can be best described if it is imagined as it would be if unwound (Fig 4). The tube is 31 mm long and is divided into three fluid-filled parallel canals, the scala vestibuli, the ductus cochlearis and the scala tympani, by two membranes, the vestibular membrane and the basilar membrane. The stapes acts as a piston and its vibrations send pressure waves up the scala vestibuli, through a narrow gap, the helicotrema, at the top of the cochlea, and down the scala tympani, finally dissipating back into the space of the middle ear by bulging the membrane of the round window. The vestibular membrane is flabby and its movements are not important, but the basilar membrane is rigid and it vibrates with the pressure waves passing through the fluid.

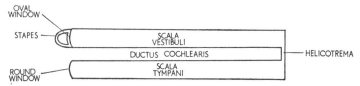

Fig 4   (a) The cochlea unwound to show the main pathway of sound. Sound waves are transmitted from the stapes, along the scala vestibuli, down the helicotrema, back through scala tympani and finally dissipated into the middle cavity at the round window

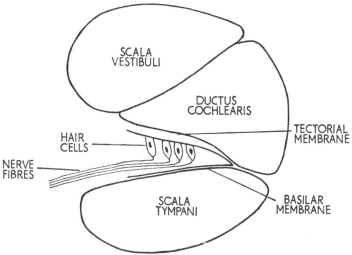

(b) Cross-section of the cochlea shows the position of the receptors

Early experiments on the ear showed that the basilar membrane was playing a very important part in the reception of pressure waves and their conversion into nerve impulses. Just above it lies the tectorial membrane and sandwiched between the two lie the hair cells, the sense cells from which the nerve fibres run. If straightened out the basilar membrane appears as a sheet, wider at one end than the other, rather like a xylophone or the strings of a piano. Examinations of the ears of people deaf to certain sounds have shown that parts of the basilar membrane were damaged. This was first noticed in a study of boilermakers' disease. Boilermakers and other men who beat or riveted metal all their working lives developed a chronic deafness to sounds of the same frequencies as the din that surrounded them all day, and it was found that the excessive noise was damaging the part of the ear that was sensitive to it. This led to a theory that the fibres of the basilar membrane were resonating like the strings of a piano. Each fibre was presumed to resonate at a particular frequency and to 'fire off' a nerve cell.

This theory was easily disproved, however, by cutting the fibres with a very fine scalpel. The cut ends did not spring apart, so the fibres could not have been under tension and therefore could not resonate. A more realistic, and more complex theory, was evolved only recently. Experiments were performed with a small piston in place of the stapes. Its movement could be controlled mechanically so that waves of a known frequency were sent up the cochlea. The waves increased in intensity and speed until they reached a maximum and then they died away. Each frequency produced by the piston reached the maximum intensity and speed at a different place along the length of the basilar membrane. High frequencies reached a maximum near the piston and low frequencies reached a maximum nearer the top of the cochlea at the other end of the membrane. Here was a straightforward way in which the analysis of frequencies could be performed mechanically by the basilar membrane. But the analysis is not simple as even a pure tone of one frequency vibrates a considerable length of membrane.

During these experiments it was found that there is a small electric charge across the basilar membrane similar to that in the nerve ending of the Pacinian corpuscle. When there are no vibrations, the charge is steady, but the passage of pressure waves causes it to oscillate. If the basilar membrane is pushed downwards, the charge increases, and if raised it decreases. The alterations to the steady charge are caused by the bending of the hair cells as the oscillating basilar membrane moves them to and fro, and they follow exactly the variations in pressure on the cochlea fluid produced by the vibrating piston, both in frequency and intensity. This is the same mechanism as that found in the microphone and Pacinian corpuscle described in Chapter One. The changing charges are called cochlear microphonics because of the similarity with the electrical changes in a microphone. They stimulate the nerve fibres and thus impulses are sent to the brain. The pattern of nerve impulses that is set in train by even a pure tone is very complex and bears no obvious relation to the frequency of that tone. The analysis by the brain of these patterns is outside the scope of this book, but it can be said that some information carried by sounds is analysed in the brain on the basis of further screening by the ears.

Ears are not only sensitive to different frequencies or loudness of sounds; they can also detect from what position the sounds are coming. Animals like deer or donkeys with a moveable pinna can locate the direction of a sound-source by swivelling their pinnas until the sound is as loud as possible. This is the same method as is used in navigation by radio-beacons. The receiving aerial is rotated until the signal from a beacon reaches maximum strength and a bearing is taken along the aerial.

One only has to watch a goat, or even a cat or dog, to see how the ears are used to pick up sound. As a car drives past the goat's field, its ears swivel round, following the car's passage along the road. A second car approaches and the goat turns one ear backwards, to concentrate on two sounds at once, and if one car backfires, the ears swing away shielding themselves from the noise in the same way that a man would stop his ears with his hands.

A simple experiment with a model of a goat's pinna will demonstrate how it increases the directional sensitivity of the ear. A model of the pinna with a microphone in it is mounted on a turntable some distance from a source of sound. As the turntable is rotated, the strength of the current from the microphone is recorded. Fig 5 shows the results expressed as a diagram. The goat's ear is most sensitive to sounds not quite in front of the animal, and it barely receives sounds from behind.

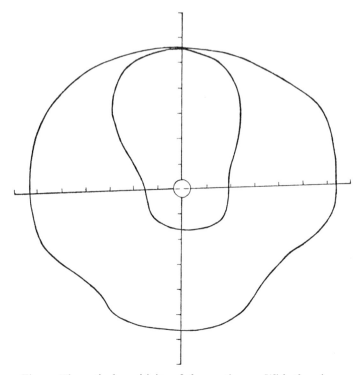

Fig 5 Theoretical sensitivity of the goat's ear. With the pinna removed the goat can hear sounds from all around with almost equal ability, but with the pinna in place the ear is most sensitive to sounds directly in front of the pinna. The scale is an arbitrary measurement of the ear's sensitivity

For a long time our pinnas have been given as examples, along with the appendix, of organs that have lost their original function and are now vestiges of their original form. At one time, it was said, they must have been like the ears of a goat or a deer. A few of us can still move our ears, but certainly not well enough to block out unpleasant sounds. Now experiments have shown that our ears are not as useless as we were led to believe. They are probably not very effective as collecting-funnels to assist in hearing faint sounds but they play an important part in detecting from which direction sounds come. The experiments on the human ear, published in 1968, are a fine example of how quite simple tests or observations can show how our previous ideas, often based on no more than speculation, can be completely wrong. The first steps in the right direction came from experiments which showed that if the human pinna was bent out of shape it was difficult to judge the position of a sound source accurately. If the pinna was just a collector of sound like an ear-trumpet, distortion would decrease the ear's ability to hear very quiet sounds, but it appeared that the pinna was doing something more.

The original experiments were limited by the amount it was possible to distort a human pinna without causing permanent injury. Neither was it possible to fit humans with pinnas of different shapes and note their effect. The problem was solved by making models of human pinnas with microphones in the ear duct. Sounds picked up by the models were then transmitted by special hearing aid-type earphones to the experimenter. Using simple models it was found that the ridges of cartilage of our pinnas act as baffles that delay the sound as it enters the ears. The amount of delay depends on the angle from which the sound comes. By comparing the difference in the time that it takes a sound to reach both ears, the brain is able to work out the position of the sound. If the sound is directly ahead or behind there is no delay; if it is to the left it takes longer to enter the right ear and so on.

There are two other methods of sound localisation, each used to a greater or lesser extent by different animals depending on the size of the animal's head and the wavelength of the sound. Even without a pinna an ear is more sensitive to sounds from one direction than another (see Fig 5). Using two ears, a sound source can be located by stereoscopic hearing in the same way as distance is judged by stereoscopic vision. The position of the sound is judged on the basis of the difference in loudness in each ear or by the difference in time it takes for the sound to reach the two ears. If the sound is above 15,000 cps the head forms a 'breakwater' which the sound waves cannot get past. Therefore the ear nearer the sound registers a much louder noise than that farther away. Alternately the difference between times of arrival of a wave at the two ears is judged. A sound wave from directly in front of the head arrives at both ears at the same time. If moved only 5° to one side the time difference is 0·00004 second and, if at right angles, 0·0005 second. With both loudness and time-difference the brain is able to discriminate, to a limited extent, between the minutely-differing signals from each ear. It can discriminate between signals 0·0001 second apart, which is a relatively large difference in time of arrival. This inefficiency can be corrected to some extent by the system of baffles in our pinnas, or by moving the head from side to side so that each ear can pinpoint the sound by the change in volume in the same way that the goat does when swivelling its pinnas. Even so human ears are not very good at locating sound and sight is usually used to help detect a source of sound.

Not so the barn owl. Until recently, owls were presumed to hunt by sight alone. They have large eyes and their eyesight seemed to be good enough to permit them to hunt in cloudy moonlight or starlight. It has now been shown by a series of experiments that barn owls can in fact locate their prey by sound alone, pouncing on moving prey with uncanny accuracy. The barn owl used for the experiments was kept in a room made as completely lightproof as a photographic darkroom. For the first tests the floor was covered with dry leaves and a mouse released from a trap. It could be heard scuffling its way through the leaves and then stop. A moment later the barn owl was heard to leave its perch, and a thud announced that it had hit the ground. The light was turned on and there was the mouse clutched in the owl's talons. Successive tests showed that the owl hit its target very much more often than it missed it, and when it did miss, the mouse escaped only narrowly.

Without careful checks these tests do not prove that the owl was detecting the mouse by the sound it made. Although sight was ruled out by the light-proofing, the owl could have been using echo-location, it could have smelt the mouse or it could have detected warmth given off by the mouse's body in the way that snakes detect warm bodies (Chapter Ten). These possibilities were eliminated by dragging a ball of paper across the floor on a string. Sure enough, the owl struck the paper so it must have been using its ears alone. For final proof the mouse was allowed to run over a bare floor on which it made no sound, and the owl was completely unable to find it.

It must not, however, be assumed from these experiments that barn owls hunt only by sound. Their eyesight is ten to a hundred times better than ours and it is very likely that they use their eyes when hunting by moonlight or at twilight. If they relied on vision they would be on short commons on overcast or moonless nights, so good hearing is an essential alternative method of finding prey. Neither can it be assumed that all owls have as good hearing, or as good vision, as barn owls. The little owl and the American burrowing owl hunt by day. It is unlikely that they use their ears very much, while their ability to see in the dark is no better than ours.

The ability of barn owls and, as is now known, of other night-hunting owls to locate their prey so accurately by hearing is partly due to the structure of their ears. The ears of birds are constructed on the same plan as ours, but the cochlea is straight instead of coiled, the three bones of the middle ear are replaced by a single bone called the columella and, usually, there is no pinna. The essential mechanism is therefore similar, but in the case of owls there are certain features that enhance its sensitivity.

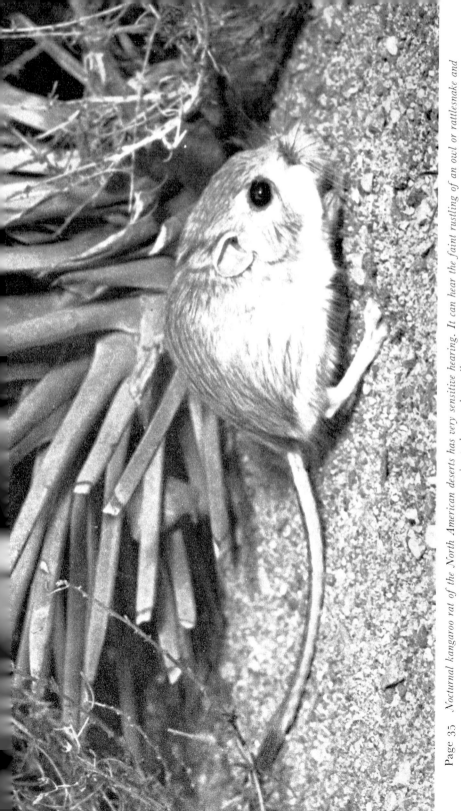

Page 35 *Nocturnal kangaroo rat of the North American deserts has very sensitive hearing. It can hear the faint rustling of an owl or rattlesnake and jump clear as they strike*

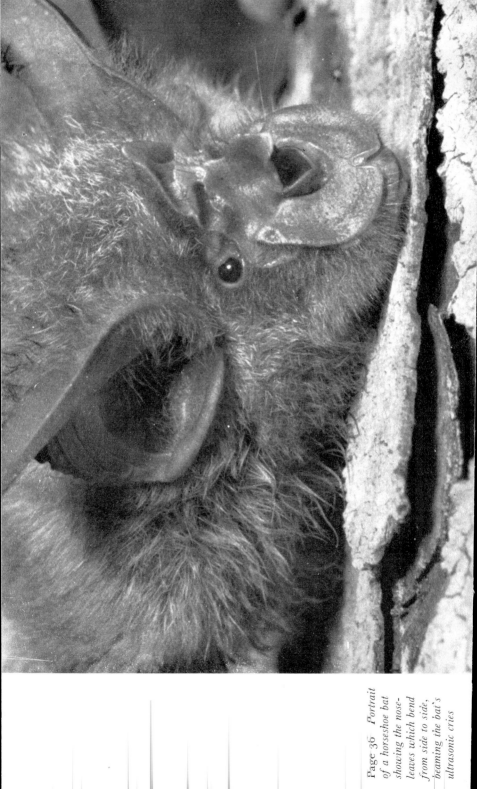

Page 36   Portrait
of a horseshoe bat
showing the nose-
leaves which bend
from side to side,
beaming the bat's
ultrasonic cries

The eardrum is large so that the columella attached to it passes on a considerable amount of sound energy to the oval window of the cochlea, which is relatively small. Thus the sound pressure is amplified a great deal, theoretically as much as forty times compared to eighteen times in our ears. The columella of most birds is attached to the centre of the eardrum, but in owls it is offset from centre and this gives a further amplification. The eardrum can be thought of as a lever. The fulcrum is at the perimeter where the drum is attached to the bone. When the eardrum vibrates, the centre bulges more than the perimeter. Movements of the eardrum then lever the columella to and fro. An offset columella, nearer the fulcrum, although not moving so far as one in the centre, is moved with greater force. In this way sound reaching an owl's ear is further concentrated before being passed to the inner ear.

Acute hearing is not enough because the owl must also know where the faint noise of the mouse is coming from. In other words, it must be able to localise the sound. It uses the same methods as ourselves, discriminating between the loudness of the sound falling on each ear and by gauging the difference in the times of arrival of a sound at each ear.

Small birds, like sparrows and garden song birds, cannot use the second method because their heads are too small. The difference in the time taken for a sound wave to reach the two ears is too minute to be registered, but as owls have larger heads, the time differences are sizeable enough to be detected.

Differences in loudness can also be used in sound localisation and experiments in which a microphone is plugged into an owl's ear show that, like the goat's, it is more sensitive to sounds from it front than from other directions. This is because barn owls have a flap of skin like a pinna around each ear which concentrates the sound. Moreover, although the ears are placed symmetrically on each side of the head, the flaps are not. Thus the difference between the volume of sounds reaching the two ears is increased and localisation is made more accurate. By moving its head about, an owl determines in which position its head must be for each ear to receive the maximum loudness from the sound source, so that in effect it is taking two bearings on the noise.

What defence does a mouse have against this almost unerring capacity of an owl to find and capture its prey? Does the owl kill indiscriminately, each mouse being as vulnerable as its neighbours, or is there a selection of prey, as one would expect if the theory of the survival of the fittest holds true? Studies of the relationships between a predator and its prey show that it is very rare for a predator to kill its prey at random or even at leisure. Most of its attacks fail and, when successful, the prey is usually young, weak or suffering from some disadvantage that puts it at risk. The mice liberated in the barn owl's room were at a definite disadvantage. They had been set free in a strange place which they had to explore. If given time to settle down they would have been difficult to capture. The experiment with the barn owl showed that an owl can hunt by hearing, but as is often true of experiments, it is misleading if applied to real life situations without discretion. In the wild, mice, voles and other small animals, do not make much noise as they move about. Every mouse lives in a system of runs through the grass or undergrowth, where it can run quietly and in comparative safety. It is possible to stand quietly by a patch of coarse grass, knowing full well that there are mice there, yet not be able to detect the slightest sign of their movement.

The mice most likely to be caught are those found away from the runs. These might be young mice that have not yet established themselves or outcasts from an overcrowded network of runs. Their only safety is to freeze at the slightest hint of danger. Yet, as was shown in the barn owl experiments, the owl may have already located the mouse. The owl has the advantage for it, too, is almost noiseless. The wing feathers of night-flying owls have soft, downy tufts along the edges, deadening the sound of the wings as the air rushes past. So the mouse's only hope is that the owl will reveal its presence by hooting. It has been said that an owl will hoot to scare mice into the open but observations show that the effect is rather the opposite. On hearing an owl hoot, a mouse freezes.

Not all small animals live in the shelter of the undergrowth where they can hide from owls. Some live in desert or semi-desert country, where cover is sparse. The outstanding feature of many small desert animals, such as the elephant shrews and jerboas of Africa and the kangaroo rats of the dry parts of the western USA and Mexico, is that they have very large auditory bullas, the dome-shaped bone behind the jaw that surrounds the middle ear. This is also a feature of larger desert animals such as the addax, the antelope that lives in the most remote parts of the Sahara desert. The large bullas have long been supposed to be linked with an acute sense of hearing, and some experiments on kangaroo rats have very neatly shown that these animals do indeed have good hearing and that this is used to warn them of the approach of enemies.

The kangaroo rat is neither a kangaroo nor a rat. It is a small mouse-like animal that looks very much like a kangaroo. It has large, powerful back legs with which it bounds across the ground, using a long tail for balance. It is nocturnal, coming out to feed on seeds which it gathers in cheek pouches and carries back to store in its burrow.

Zoologists have studied the kangaroo rat largely because it is able to live on dry food without drinking, but our interest is in its large, paper-thin ear bones that form the middle ears. Together they make a volume greater than the brain itself. Within the bullas are found some of the same adaptations giving increased sensitivity that are seen in the barn owl's ear: the eardrum is large and the stapes fits into a very small oval window. A comparison of the areas of the eardrum and the oval window showed that sounds are magnified nearly 100 times by the middle ear.

The large volume of the bullas also serves to increase sensitivity. This was tested by anaesthetising kangaroo rats and carefully inserting minute electrodes into their cochleas. Sounds of varying frequency were played to them and the cochlear microphonics produced were picked up by the electrodes. The kangaroo rats were found to be particularly sensitive to sounds between 1,000 and 3,000 cps. When the spaces in the bullas were filled up, the sensitivity of the ears was very much reduced although the rats still responded to sounds over the same range of frequency.

The large cavities of the bullas must, therefore, improve the hearing of the kangaroo rat. The reason for this appears to be that in a normal-sized middle ear the vibrations of the eardrum are reduced by the pressure of air in the bulla behind the drum. If the bulla is small a movement inwards by the eardrum quickly builds up pressure behind, counteracting the movement, but if the bulla is large there is no such counteraction and the eardrum can vibrate freely. This is especially true for sounds of lower frequency. Low frequency vibrations cause more exaggerated movements of the eardrum, and it is to the lower frequencies that kangaroo rats are most sensitive, differing in this way from most other small mammals, which are especially sensitive to sounds well above 3,000 cps.

The next step in these experiments was to find out whether the extreme sensitivity of a kangaroo rat's ears was of any value to the animal. Were they sensitive enough to warn it of predators? Kangaroo rats are active at night so they run the danger of being killed by night-hunters. In the deserts of the USA these include owls and rattlesnakes. So experiments were carried out like those already described with the barn owl and the mice, only on this occasion kangaroo rats were pitted against a barn owl and a rattlesnake. Both can hunt in the dark, the barn owl by listening, as shown, and the rattlesnake by detecting the body heat of its prey. The kangaroo rat was first placed in a cage with the owl. By using red light, which the rats cannot see, it was possible to watch their behaviour as if in complete darkness. Each time the owl pounced, the kangaroo rat jumped out of the way. In a quite spectacular way, just as the apparently unaware kangaroo rat was about to be caught, it leaped straight up and landed a foot or so away, leaving the owl clutching the ground where it had been standing. The same happened when the snake struck. Finally, to prove the value of the large bullas, these were blocked up with plasticine. Now the kangaroo rats were completely ignorant of impending doom until too late.

There was one last question. The wings of owls are muffled by special downy feathers so that they can fly silently. In view of this, how does the kangaroo rat detect an owl? While these experiments were being made, a tape-recorder was being run with the volume turned as high as possible. Careful analysis of the tapes showed that as the owl struck there was a faint whisper of sound with frequencies up to 1,200 cps. Similarly the snake produced sound with frequencies up to 2,000 cps as it struck. These frequencies lie in the range to which the ear of the kangaroo rat is most sensitive, although the sounds could only be detected at the very limit of the tape recorder's sensitivity.

The development of the powers of hearing of the owl and the kangaroo rat is the outcome of natural selection and can be thought of as analogous to human conflict; one nation produces a weapon and its adversaries have to find a counter to it or perish. Throughout the history of war there has been a continual process of inventing weapons and tactics, then developing their antidotes. The barn owl developed a method of finding its prey and avoiding giving itself away. Its prey learnt to keep hidden or develop an early-warning system. None of the systems are perfect, sometimes a mouse is too slow and sometimes an owl goes hungry, so both predator and prey are balanced against one another.

CHAPTER THREE

Recognition sounds

The buzz of the bee and the chirp of the grasshopper are familiar noises on a warm day—just pleasant summer sound effects, to human ears. And indeed, until recently there appeared to be no more significance to the buzz of a bee than in the noise of an aircraft engine. But research has revealed that the noises some insects make with their wings are a vital means of communication. They serve for instance as courtship signals; and in the case of the bee the buzz of its wings, beating as many as 200 times a second, can augment the well-known 'waggle dance' (Chapter Seven) and communicate the position of a source of nectar. Other insects have more elaborate ways of producing sound. The 'chirps' or stridulation of grasshoppers and crickets are also courtship songs but are produced by rubbing a leg to and fro along the serrated edge of a wing or by rubbing two wings together.

It is difficult to conceive of animals as primitive as insects indulging in courtship, especially with 'songs', but the rituals of courtship not only constitute the method by which animals of different sexes are brought together and often by which they are stimulated to breeding condition, but also ensure that an animal mates only with one of its own kind and not with a close relation. These factors are as important to insects as they are to birds and mammals, and it is only since the development of apparatus with which to eavesdrop on insects that the significance of their behaviour has become clear.

If insects make sounds, it seems likely that they must also be able to detect them, that is, they must have organs of hearing.

At the moment quite a few insects are known to have hearing organs and others may be discovered as more insects are studied in detail. The organs range from simple hairs protruding from the hard skin of the insect and attached at the base to a single sense cell, to complex structures that resemble the ears of vertebrates. The resemblance in this case is, however, confined to appearance. It is not strictly correct to speak of insect ears, as their hearing organs operate in a different manner to vertebrate ears and they are sensitive to different properties of sound.

In the early part of this century our knowledge was extended by the entomologist, Regen, who conducted some experiments with crickets. He put a male cricket under a glass bowl and found that nearby females took no notice of it although it was clearly visible. When, however, a microphone was placed near the male and its chirping was relayed over a telephone, the females gathered around the loudspeaker. So the females were attracted to the sound and not to the sight of the male. The experiments also shed light on the mechanism by which crickets hear. It was found that the females were attracted to the loudspeaker even when the sounds coming from it were so distorted that to human ears they seemed quite unlike the chirping of a cricket. Other insects were also able to recognise sounds that meant nothing to the human ear.

The puzzle was solved some years later when a method of recording the impulses travelling along the nerve leading from an insect's hearing organ was devised. The exact response of the organ to a particular sound could be recorded so that it was possible to tell to which property of the sound the organ was responding. The method of recording is essentially very simple: a locust, cricket or other large insect is anaesthetised and a fine wire electrode attached to the nerve running from one hearing organ. The impulses passing down the nerve are amplified and fed into an oscilloscope. This is very like the arrangement used to record the sensitivity of the kangaroo rat's hearing described in the previous chapter. Sounds of different frequencies were played to the anaesthetised insect and the pattern of response recorded. Different insects are sensitive to a greatly varying range of frequencies. Crickets are sensitive to frequencies between 250 and 10,000 cps, grasshoppers to those between 800 and 45,000 cps, well into the ultrasonic range, while certain night-flying moths, of the family Noctuidae, respond to sounds with frequencies of up to 150,000 cps. The importance of the ability to hear ultrasonic frequencies by these moths will become clear in the next chapter where it is shown that they are able to detect the ultrasonic pulses used by bats in finding their prey.

Records obtained from the oscilloscope show that the nervous response bears no relation to the sounds falling on the auditory organ, except that they parallel the intensity. As the sound becomes louder there is a greater frequency of nerve impulses flowing along the nerve. There is no echoing of the frequency of the sound as there is in the cochlear microphonics in our ears. The hearing organs of locusts, for instance, were found to be very sensitive to sounds of about 8,000 cps, but the nervous responses to such sounds did not follow any pattern. Yet Regen's experiments had shown that insects were able to distinguish between different sounds, as female crickets were attracted only to males of their own species. This meant that there must be some feature of the sound that the auditory organs can analyse and that the crickets can recognise. Further oscilloscope experiments showed that the property of sound to which the insects were sensitive was pulse modulation.

A sound of pure tone or constant frequency is called a carrier wave (Fig 6a). Without changing the frequency, the amplitude or intensity may be varied. Moreover, it may be varied at regular intervals, so that the amplitude varies at a certain frequency independent of the carrier wave (Fig 6b). Therefore there is an amplitude frequency superimposed on the carrier wave frequency. The former is called the modulation frequency of the carrier wave. In Fig 6b, there is a modulation frequency of 400 cps on a carrier wave of 1,000 cps. The modulation need not be the rhythmic variation of amplitude shown in Fig 6b, it can be a cutting of the carrier wave into distinct pulses (Fig 6c).

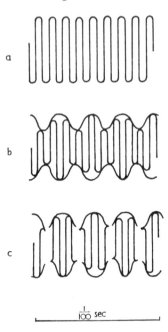

Fig 6 Frequency modulation. (a) shows unmodulated sound waves with a frequency of 1,000 cps. In (b) a modulation wave of 400 cps is superimposed on the 1,000 cps carrier wave. The modulation wave in (c) has been 'chopped' to make it pulse modulated

This is called pulse modulation. Radio telegraphy is a form of pulse modulation in which the carrier wave generated in the transmitter is modulated by a key into the series of dots and dashes that make up the morse code.

Returning to insects, their sensitivity to pulse modulation shows that they are communicating by a sort of morse code. The chirping of the male cricket consists of a pattern of pulse modulation that has a special meaning to females of its own species. When the auditory organ of an anaesthetised insect is stimulated by a sound with a frequency of 8,000 cps, no particular pattern of nervous impulses is produced. But when this sound is modulated, with frequencies up to 300 cps, the nerves send bursts of impulses corresponding to the modulating frequencies. The

45

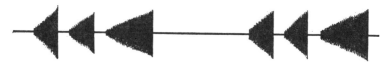

Fig 7   Simplified diagram of two 'phases' of a cricket song

pattern of these bursts is unaffected by variations of the carrier frequencies.

This explains why the female crickets in Regen's experiments responded to the distorted sounds coming over the telephone. Our ears are sensitive to changes of frequency in the carrier wave, while crickets are sensitive only to the modulated frequencies. The telephone was distorting the carrier waves but not the modulations, so to an insect there was no difference.

The difference in hearing ability between insects and men lies in the construction of the hearing organs. A hearing organ detects either variations in pressure set up by sound waves on a membrane or the amount it is displaced by the waves. The vertebrate ear is a pressure detector, consisting essentially of a box, the middle ear, with a stretched membrane, the eardrum, over one end. The pressure is kept the same on either side of the membrane by means of a valve, the eustachian tube which opens into the back of the mouth. The 'popping' in our ears when going up in an aeroplane or even driving down a steep hill is caused by the eustachian tube opening to let air in or out and so equalise the pressure on the eardrum. As the middle ear is, therefore, a closed box with a steady pressure inside the

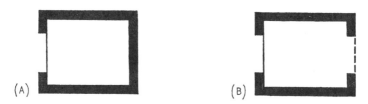

(A)   (B)

Fig 8   The essential differences between (a) vertebrate ear (pressure sensitive) and (b) insect hearing organ (displacement sensitive). The former is a closed box, the latter is open at one end

membrane, minute fluctuations of pressure on the outside, when sound waves fall on it, cause the membrane to be pushed in or drawn out and the pressure changes to be transmitted to the inner ear.

The hearing organs of grasshoppers, crickets, moths and their relatives are displacement detectors. They are called tympanic organs after the drumlike membrane, but by comparison with the vertebrate ear the barrel of the drum is open at one end (Fig 8). When a sound strikes the membrane there is little difference in pressure on either side of it, and the membrane therefore moves in accordance with the displacement of the air. The sense organs are at the base of the membrane and record the amount it bends. Hairs and antennae that are hearing organs work in essentially the same way, except that there is no box around them. Because pressure acts equally in all directions a single vertebrate ear cannot detect the direction of a sound

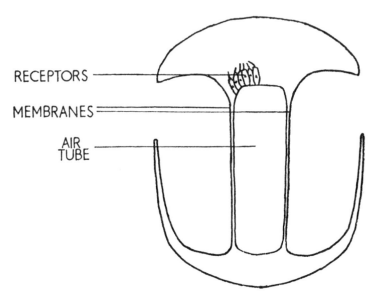

RECEPTORS

MEMBRANES

AIR
TUBE

Fig 9 Simplified hearing organ on the foreleg of a grasshopper. The air tube which opens to the outside corresponds to the box in Fig 8 (b)

without a pinna, but displacement is directional, the maximum displacement occurring when the membrane is facing the sound source, and insect hearing organs can, therefore, detect direction. This means that an insect can tell where a sound is coming from with only one hearing organ, and blocking one organ does little to impede a female cricket locating a singing male.

It has been suggested that the ability of insects to locate sound is assisted by leg movements. Insect hearing organs are found on many different parts of the body. Those of grasshoppers and crickets are on the 'knee' joint of the front legs, a ridiculous place for a sense organ of a human but useful to the grasshopper when one considers that the function of its hearing organs is to steer the legs so that the animal moves towards a sound. As the legs move to and fro they swing through an arc so that the hearing organs scan both sides of the animal. Each organ is very sensitive to sounds coming from certain angles, so as the legs swing round there is an outburst or falling off of nerve impulses as they pass a sound source and the central nervous system compares this with the position of the legs and so finds out the direction from which the sound is coming.

There is more to the songs of crickets and grasshoppers than was demonstrated through Regen's telephone experiments. Firstly, only virgin females are attracted by the songs of males; fertilised females ignore them. Furthermore, each species has a variety of songs, for different situations. Some species may have a dozen songs, a fact once appreciated by the Chinese who kept crickets and even bred them specially for their songs. The normal song of crickets can be heard from a lone male or as a chorus of several males. It serves to attract the females and bring the males together so that the females may find them more easily. In the presence of a female a male sings a 'serenade', followed by the courtship song which immediately precedes mating. During mating he may sing another song if the female gets restless and, if disturbed by another male, he sings a 'rival's duet'.

Apart from courtship and mating songs, crickets and many

other insects have alarm or warning calls, usually a loud noise emitted when they are touched, which may scare enemies away. There is one fly that, for its protection, appears to imitate the buzzing of a wasp, so deceiving enemies into thinking that it is poisonous. It is quite common for harmless insects to mimic the colour patterns of poisonous insects. A visit to the clumps of cow parsley growing around the edges of woods in summer will reveal on the flowerheads swarms of hoverflies striped yellow and black in imitation of bees and wasps. After eating a few poisonous insects, birds learn to avoid ones with yellow and black stripes, including the non-poisonous ones. One of these hoverflies has gone one step further, by mimicking the sound of a particular wasp. The wasp's wingbeat is 150 per second while that of the fly is 147 per second, a difference undetectable to the birds that are likely to eat it.

The courtship songs of crickets and their relatives are produced by parts of the body being rubbed together rhythmically, or, in the case of cicadas, by a pair of drums called tymbals which are rapidly drawn in and out by powerful muscles so that they click in a similar way to a biscuit-tin lid being pressed in with a finger.

Other insects, like the honeybee, communicate by the natural sound of the wingbeats, the engine-note as it were; each species of insect having a distinct note by which it can be identified in the same way that during World War II aircraft were identified by their engines long before they came into sight. In the insect world there is a wide variation in the rate of wingbeat, from the 5 per second of some large butterflies to over 1,000 per second of minute biting midges. The wings of wasps beat 110 times per second, those of houseflies 190 times per second, while mosquitoes' wings beat at around 500 times per second. The wingbeats produce waves in the air in the same way as the vibration of a tuning fork. At the higher rates of wingbeat the frequencies of the waves are audible to us as a constant buzz or hum. In many instances the noise is merely fortuitous and plays no part in the life of the insect, but in some insects it has been put to use as a medium for communication, as is the case with the elaborate songs of the crickets and grasshoppers.

The first person to investigate the role of wingbeat sound in insect communication was the inventor Sir Hiram Maxim. He is better known as an engineer and for his invention of the Vickers Maxim machine gun but he was one of those people with a wide knowledge and a sense of curiosity that led him to investigate anything unusual. In 1878 Maxim erected a line of electric lamps to illuminate the grounds of the Grand Union Hotel in Saratoga Springs, New York. Part of the mechanism used for producing a suitable electric current was a transformer that vibrated producing a humming note. One evening Maxim noticed that large numbers of mosquitoes had gathered around the transformer. While another man perhaps would have noticed this only as a matter of passing interest, Maxim stopped to examine the mosquitoes more closely. He recognised them as males because of their feathery antennae, the antennae of female mosquitoes being clublike with very few hairs. The next step was to watch while the lamps were turned on in the evening. As soon as the humming started all the male mosquitoes in the vicinity turned towards the source of the noise and flew to it. Maxim then had the idea that the pair of feathery antennae on the head of each male mosquito acted as 'ears' and that the mosquitoes were flying to the lamp because it was making a noise like the humming of a female mosquito. This theory was put to the test with a tuning fork that mimicked the female mosquito's hum. Each time Maxim struck the fork near a male mosquito the latter turned to face the vibrating fork and raised its antennae. In this way Maxim showed that male mosquitoes are attracted to the humming of the females and that the sound of his transformer had been misleading them. Maxim confessed to being no naturalist, yet by keen observation and astute reasoning, reinforced by a simple experiment, he had demonstrated the role of sound in the life of mosquitoes. The story is a very good example of the way scientific investigation should be carried out, except in its ending. A scientific journal rejected the account as being too silly to be worth publishing. Instead, Maxim published his findings in a letter to *The Times*.

Another seventy years passed before the humming of female mosquitoes came under a more detailed scrutiny. Of the many species of mosquito, one in particular was selected for examination. This was *Aëdes aegypti*, the mosquito that carries yellow fever. If mosquitoes could be attracted by sound it was thought that their numbers might possibly be reduced and the disease controlled by 'baiting' traps with the humming of a female mosquito. The first experiments added further evidence to support Maxim's conclusions. Mosquitoes mate while in flight so to study the behaviour of the males a female was glued to a fine wire and suspended in mid-air. While she beat her wings male mosquitoes flew to her and mated with her. But if her wingbeats stopped, the males immediately lost interest and would fly past her as if she did not exist. Further experiments showed that males were attracted from distances of up to 10 in, a limit that unfortunately eliminated the possibility of luring mosquitoes by sound as a means of controlling their numbers in the wild.

As Maxim had suspected, the males' antennae are the sense organs of hearing. Female yellow fever mosquitoes beat their wings at 450–600 cps, producing an audible noise of this frequency. Tests with tuning forks vibrating at different frequencies showed that the males responded to sounds with frequencies between 300 and 800 cps, more than covering the sounds made by the females. A close examination showed that within these frequencies the males' antennae vibrated in time to the vibrations of the tuning forks. If blobs of glue were placed on the tip of the antennae, weighting them so that they could not vibrate, the males failed to heed the siren call of the females, thus demonstrating that the antennae are indeed the auditory organs of the mosquitoes. The feathery structure acts like the aerial of the Jodrell Bank radio telescope, presenting a large surface area to receive the incoming signals. The vibrations are transmitted down the centre shaft of the antenna to the base where they stimulate a sense organ called Johnston's organ. The antennae

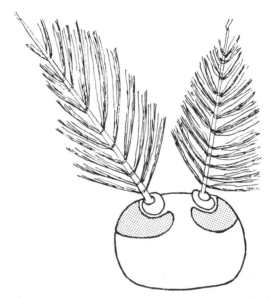

Fig 10   The feathery antennae of the mosquito vibrate in time to sound waves and their movements stimulate Johnston's organs in the bulbs at their bases

are vibrating like the membrane of the cricket's hearing organ, reacting to displacement by sound waves. The shaft of the antenna articulates in the bulb-shaped base by means of a flexible membrane. Attached to the membrane are sense cells that register the amount of bending and pass on the information to nerve fibres leading to the brain.

The attraction of the males by the female mosquito is beautifully simple: as she flies about the hum produced by the female's wingbeats guides the males to her, but the males are not attracted to each other because their wingbeats are too fast to stimulate each other's antennae. This is, however, not the whole story, which is even neater. Male mosquitoes do not become sexually mature until a few days after they have emerged from the pupae. During this time the hairs on the antennae lie almost flat along the shaft and the humming of a female will not be sensed unless she is very close. As a result the young males do

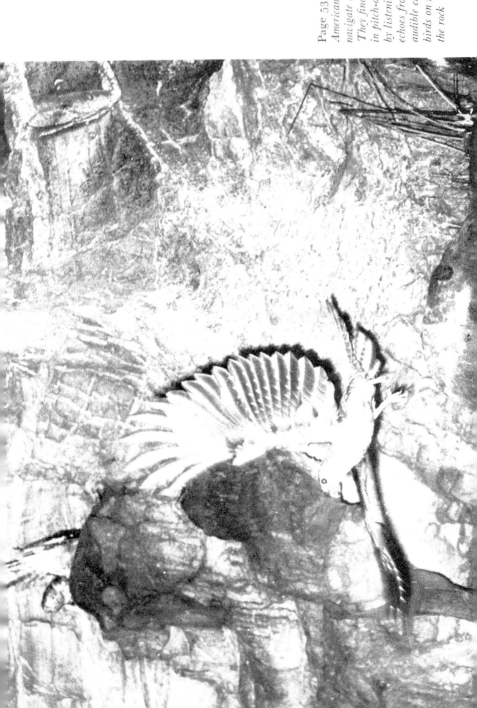

Page 53 South American oilbirds navigate by sonar. They find their way in pitch-dark caves by listening to the echoes from their audible clicks. Note birds on nest, behind the rock

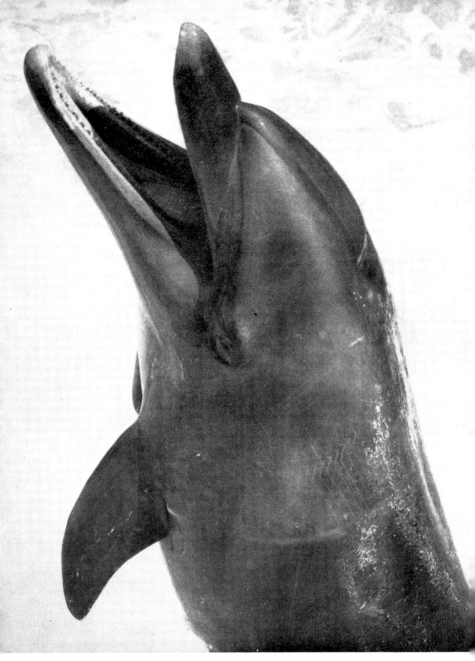

Page 54   *The 'melon' lies between the beak and blowhole of this dolphin and focuses the ultrasonic calls produced in the blowhole. A line of sensory pits can just be seen on the beak. Each pit contains the remains of a whisker and may be used to detect vibrations in the water*

not waste energy chasing females to no purpose and only start courting when their antennae have fluffed out and they are mature. The females are also infertile when young and they are ignored by the males because, until mature, their wingbeats are slow and produce a hum of too low a frequency to attract the males. This is a very clear example of how an animal's behaviour can be carefully regulated to its best advantage. Changes in organs of movement and hearing are timed by simple processes so that the sexes are brought together for breeding at the right moment. As the changes are physical, needing no organisation to control them, there is no need for systems of complicated nervous or hormonal control. This is a great advantage to an insect whose nerve cells are comparatively large compared to ours. It has only limited space in its body for nerve tissue so 'control systems' that organise its behaviour must be kept to a minimum.

With the fruit flies, courtship is reversed, the male singing to the female. Fruit flies are the small flies that can usually be seen wherever fruit is stored. They are also attracted to wine or beer glasses and these are the small flies that one sometimes has to rescue from these beverages. In appearance they are like miniature yellowish or brownish house flies that fly slowly and heavily with abdomens hanging down as though they can only just remain airborne.

There is one further important difference between the fruit fly's courtship and that of the mosquito. The humming of a female mosquito may attract males of other species, cross-breeding being avoided since the male is able to confirm that she is the right female by smell. Fruit flies make sure that mating takes place between a pair of the same species not only by smell but also often by sight and hearing, the female deciding who is right for her.

There are about 2,000 species of fruit **fly** and some are so similar that the differences can only be detected under a high-power microscope. Yet very similar fruit flies can be kept together without cross-breeding taking place. Courtship takes place on the ground and, unlike the yellow fever mosquitoes, their antics can quite easily be watched, although only a few of the 2,000 species have been studied. A male fruit fly courts a female with quite an elaborate ceremonial, after which she will accept or reject him. First the male walks up to the female and taps her abdomen with his forefeet. Then he stands behind her or circles around, all the time displaying with his wings, flicking or vibrating them. It seems that the courtship stimulates the female and enables her to distinguish a male of her own species from any other. If she is not yet mature, or if her suitor is of the wrong kind, she buzzes very loudly, an answer to his courting that is firmly negative and results in his discouraged departure.

The pattern of courtship differs between species. Some rely on smell, others on sight or sound, or a combination of the three. In a few of the species investigated, sound plays the major part, and a female will only accept a male if he sings the right tune. Close examination of the wing displays of these fruit flies shows that the songs produced by them are almost constant within a species, each species producing a signature tune that is sufficiently different from other very closely related species to prevent inter-breeding.

Recording the songs is not easy. Fruit flies are only about $\frac{1}{8}$ in long and the sounds they produce are weak, so it is no use holding a microphone near them in the hope of getting a recording. The only practical way of recording fruit flies is to replace the gauze guard of a very sensitive microphone with a small perspex cage. The fruit flies are then free to run round actually on the diaphragm of the microphone. Elaborate precautions have to be taken to prevent outside noises drowning the fruit fly songs. One experimental set-up consisted of a series of plasterboard boxes, like a nest of saucepans, with glass wool between them. The boxes, with the cage and microphone nestling in them, stood on two paving stones with soft rubber balls sandwiched between them, and the whole stood on an inflated motorcar inner tube. These precautions were comparable with those in the story of the princess and the pea, yet the researchers still found that it was necessary to work at night or over the weekend to prevent outside noises spoiling their recordings.

Fruit fly songs are similar in quality to those of crickets. They are pulse modulated, that is they are made up of bursts of sound waves, which are produced by the wings beating. Some fruit flies open both wings during the courtship display, while others open only one. If the wings are fully opened the frequency of the wingbeat is the same as that used in flying. This is about 200 cps in most species and is very similar to the frequency of the waves in the song. Other fruit flies court with their wings only partly opened, so that they beat faster and produce a higher-pitched sound.

Three components of the pulse modulated sounds produced by fruit flies are variable: the number of waves in each burst, the time between bursts and the frequency of the waves in the bursts. The number of waves varies very little between species. The other two components are constant within a species but vary considerably between species. Two almost identical species of fruit fly are *Drosophila pseudoobscura* and *Drosophila persimilis*. In the laboratory they can be induced to mate and to produce hybrid offspring. This means that they can only just be classed as separate species, as the usual definition of a species is a group of animals that cannot mate with others outside the group to produce fertile offspring. In the wild the two would not normally mate and it is likely that it is the time lapse between bursts in their songs that keeps them apart. The time between bursts is the modulation frequency, to which insect hearing organs are particularly sensitive, and it is five times greater in the songs of male *D. pseudoobscura* than in *D. persimilis*.

Fruit flies are one of the commonest of laboratory animals. The large number of species and the rapid rate of breeding, together with certain features of their tissues has made them the standard animal for studies on genetics. Because they are readily available they are also used for other investigations, such as the ones described above. Most insects, however, are studied with a more practical end in view. As a group, insects do far more damage to human health and property than any other animals. Every new crop soon acquires its insect pests and today's rapid means of communication have resulted in the inevitable spread of insect pests around the world, so that many laboratories and field stations are devoted wholly to finding ways of eradicating these insects. Some projects aim at attracting insects to a poison as being a safer method than spreading poison around in the hope that the insects will eventually fall foul of it. Some success has been obtained by luring insects by smell (see Chapter Eight), but the use of specific sounds like those used to attract crickets or mosquitoes has as yet been unsuccessful. As has already been indicated male yellow fever mosquitoes are attracted by the sound of a female but only if she is less than 10 in away. The obvious solution of recording the sound made by the female and playing it back through an amplifier is unfortunately ruled out since for some reason as yet unexplained, an amplified sound of a female mosquito drives the males away. However, research on insect sounds is still in its infancy and another more promising line of attack is described in the next chapter.

CHAPTER FOUR

Animal sonar systems

Bats are ugly: their faces are misshapen, their wings wrinkled and leathery and to many people they are the objects of a deeply-rooted fear, often prompted by warnings that a bat will fly into your hair. To say that this is unlikely and that there is no proof that bats get tangled in people's hair, as one writer did, is to invite a deluge of mail relating first-hand experiences. And yet why should bats fly into anyone's hair? It is now common knowledge that they have a system of echolocation or sonar that enables them to avoid obstacles and catch their food in complete darkness. By emitting high-frequency, ultrasonic squeaks and listening for the incredibly faint echoes, bats are able to navigate with uncanny accuracy, and even avoid wires, almost as fine as strands of hair, placed in their path.

It is easy enough to watch bats hunting and to see that they are finding their prey with remarkable skill. They are more common than is generally supposed and can often be seen silhouetted against the sky at dusk, flitting around in a vague, seemingly purposeless fashion, and then suddenly darting away and swerving off before returning to their original circling. Each sudden spurt indicates an insect being chased, and probably caught. If the bat is hunting over open ground its prowess can be tested by throwing small pebbles in the air. I found the perfect place for this while on holiday in Sussex. On the outskirts of the village there was a municipal rubbish tip. At dusk this became the hunting ground for more than fifty bats. It was an odd experience, terrifying to some no doubt, to have these bats wheeling about one's head, sometimes only a foot away. By throwing a pebble in the air it was possible to attract a bat's attention, causing it to swerve around and follow the path of the falling stone, spiralling down after it, then sheering off and resuming its flight. Obviously the bat had detected the pebble by its sonar but it did not make the mistake of catching and swallowing the stone. On what basis did it decide that the stone was inedible? It could be that its sonar was so sensitive that at close quarters it could tell the difference between an insect and a pebble, but in that case one would not expect it to have followed the pebble at all. A more probable answer is that the bat finally discovers whether an object is edible by smell or by the sound that it makes.

On another occasion I was able to watch a bat actually catching its prey. Bats sometimes come out in daylight, usually in late afternoon. This bat, however, appeared several days running in brilliant mid-day sun. It flew back and forth over the lawn and for the first time I was able to see a flying bat as more than a silhouette. Its body was brown and furry and its wings almost transparent in the sunshine. While I was watching it, a butterfly came flying across the lawn at a height of about 50 ft. The bat chased after it, repeatedly swooping down, but at each attack the butterfly dodged and the bat swept past. Eventually the butterfly escaped into some trees. The bat was probably a youngster, inexperienced in hunting, and this was confirmed by its behaviour when I threw pebbles in the air to lure it down for a closer look. Like the bats over the rubbish tip this bat spiralled down after the pebble, but then the pebble suddenly disappeared. The bat had caught it, and only a few seconds later released it. The pebble had been caught in the interfemoral membrane, the flap of skin that runs between the hind legs of bats and acts as an extra wing surface. Or this is what I assumed to have happened, because the action was too quick to follow with the naked eye.

The sequence of events enacted in catching insects has been studied by photography, with a cine camera and by using multi-flash. In multi-flash photography a still camera is used in conjunction with a flash unit that can be fired very rapidly. The shutter of the camera is opened and the flash triggered. Each flash produces an image, so that one plate bears a succession of images taken at very short intervals.

Bats were released into a room where they caught fruit flies or butterflies, or even mealworms shot from a spring-operated gun. Photographs showed that small insects like fruit flies were sometimes caught in the mouth but more usually insects were caught in the interfemoral membrane. Just before the bat intercepts an insect the legs are brought forward so that the interfemoral membrane forms a scoop. The insect is swept up and picked out with the mouth by bringing the head down into the scoop. If the bat is slightly off course the insect is hooked towards the scoop by one wing. The efficiency of the method is shown by the bat's ability to catch up to fourteen fruit flies in a minute, while photographs showed that they were sometimes able to catch two fruit flies within half a second.

The story of the bat's 'radar' is a favourite in those 'Nature thought of it first' articles that periodically crop up in magazines. About thirty years ago the technique of radiolocation or radar was developed. By this method radio waves are bounced off distant objects and the echoes picked up and analysed to ascertain the objects' positions and movement. Some forty million years previously the bats had developed a similar system, but using sound waves instead of radio waves. With their 'radar', or sonar as it is better known, they are able to detect, track down and capture flying insects in complete darkness. As radar technology has advanced so the bats' sonar has become better understood and its mechanism seems more and more incredible. Far from being the crude system illustrated by the diagrams accompanying the 'Nature thought of it first' stories of sound waves travelling from the bat's mouth to the insect and back to the bat's ear, the mechanism was found to be so very intricate that one feels a sense of awe at the beauty and subtlety of nature —one might even call it cleverness—that the simple stories could never convey. The workings of the bat's sonar has not been completely unravelled, but we are constantly finding that bats employ techniques that are being developed in the most advanced radar sets, although the mechanism is packed into a small part of a tiny brain.

The first step in the discovery of bats' sonar was made by an Italian scientist, Lazaro Spallanzani. In 1793 Spallanzani caught some bats in a belltower, blinded them and released them some distance away. The blind bats flew back to their roosts in the tower, and even caught insects on the way. Meanwhile a Swiss naturalist had plugged the ears of some bats and found that they were incapable of navigating and merely blundered about helplessly. It therefore became apparent that bats needed their ears, but not their eyes, to find their way about and catch insects. Spallanzani could only suggest that they could somehow 'see' with their ears and it was not until 1920 that the idea was put forward that they might be using sound of frequencies too high for us to hear—ultrasonics. Then in 1938 Donald Griffin, working at Harvard University, performed a long series of experiments that showed how bats were able to avoid obstacles by ultrasonic echolocation. Later experiments showed how insects were tracked down and caught.

The ultrasonic cries of bats were demonstrated for the first time when Griffin took a cage of bats to the laboratory of Professor Pierce who had invented a machine that converted high frequency sound to lower frequency wavelengths audible to the human ear. As soon as this 'bat detector' was directed at the cage, the loudspeaker erupted with a cacophony of rattles and crackles. Shortly afterwards, Griffin joined up with a physiologist, Galambos, to perform the basic experiments that show how acute is the bats' sonar. Curtains of wires suspended 1 ft apart were arranged in a room where the bats were allowed to fly about, and the number of times a bat hit a wire as it flew through a curtain was counted. Individual bats varied in their ability to avoid the wires. None was perfect but some were extremely adept. When the wires were 1 mm thick the bats only touched them two times out of ten. As finer wires were substituted their scores decreased but even when the wires were 0·3 mm thick the bats still dodged them more often than they hit them. Only when the wires were 0·07 mm thick, about the diameter of human hair, did the bats fail completely to locate them. To hear echoes from these fine wires must need astonishingly acute hearing and another test showed that a bat can still detect wires even when its ears are being bombarded with ultrasonic noise from loudspeakers on either side. Only when the wires were reduced to a diameter of $\frac{1}{2}$ mm did the bats fail to detect them. Although the loudspeakers were blanketing the room with sound waves as loud as the sounds the bats were emitting, they were still able to hear the echoes 2,000 times fainter coming back from the wires. This is rather like hearing someone whispering through the roar of a football crowd.

In the thirty years following these original experiments, Griffin has elucidated many of the mechanisms by which bats are able to avoid fine wires and to catch insects. He has not been alone in the field and there is now a vast amount of information about the mechanism of echolocation based on laboratory studies. Armed with this information and freed from the laboratory by the development of sophisticated lightweight apparatus biologists are now studying bats in their natural surroundings to find out how the mechanisms are used in everyday life. Among the first mechanisms to be studied were those of sound emission and hearing, the all-important physiological processes involved in echolocation.

The commonest bats in Europe and most of North America belong to the family of vesper bats. The pipistrelle or flittermouse, *die Fledermaus* in German, that most people will have seen at dusk is a vesper bat. The two species that Griffin used in his experiments, called the little brown bat and the big brown bat, are also vespers. Photographs of vespers show that they fly with their mouths open so it is reasonable to conclude that the ultrasonic pulses are emitted through their mouths. A crude but effective experiment confirmed this. When a bat's mouth was held underwater no ultrasonics could be detected, but when the

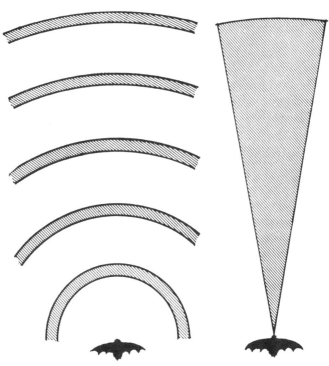

Fig 11 (left) Short, spreading impulses of a vespertilionid bat. (right) Long, beamed impulse from a horseshoe bat sweeps from side to side

rest of the body was submerged, leaving the mouth above water, ultrasonics and audible protests were amply in evidence. The ultrasonics are produced by a very much enlarged larynx or voice box but how the continuous train of extremely short squeaks are produced is not known.

The vesper bats have come to be seen as the 'standard bats' but by no means all bats use sonar. The tropical fruit bats do not, for instance, and not all species emit ultrasonics through the mouth. Horseshoe bats fly with their mouths closed, emitting ultrasonics through their nostrils. The bats I had seen over the rubbish tip in Sussex were mainly greater horseshoe bats, together with a few lesser horseshoes. These are the two common

European species and can be distinguished from other bats by the two strange fleshy growths around their nostrils that together look rather like a horseshoe. Other families of bats have even more bizarre and indescribably ugly structures on their faces.

The noseleaves, as these particular structures are called, play an important part in the emission of ultrasonics. While a horseshoe bat is in flight its noseleaves are continually in motion, bending from side to side. They act as reflectors, concentrating the ultrasonics into a narrow beam about 20° wide which sweeps from side to side of the bat's path. By contrast, the ultrasonics of vesper bats are emitted as pulses that spread in all directions, although they are most intense when recorded from directly in front of the bat.

There is a fundamental difference between the emissions of vesper bats and horseshoe bats. Pulses of vespers are frequency modulated. In each pulse there is a frequency sweep, the frequency changing rapidly from high to low. The horseshoe bats, on the other hand, emit pulses of almost constant frequency. Each pulse is comparatively long, lasting for as much as 100/ 1,000 sec or 100 milliseconds. They are sometimes of sufficiently low enough frequency to be audible to us, when they can be heard as a faint ticking like that of a watch.

The returning echoes are extremely faint, perhaps 2,000 times as weak as the original pulses. This sets the bat's ears two prob-

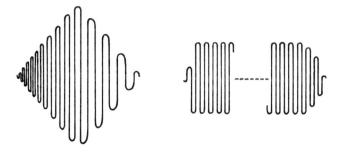

Fig 12   (left) The pulse of a vespertilionid bat changes in frequency, denoted by the spacing of the vertical lines, and loudness. (right) The pulse of a horseshoe bat is steady in frequency and loudness

lems: to register a very faint echo, far fainter than anything human ears can detect, and not to be deafened by the outgoing pulse that is emitted only a few thousandths of a second before the echo returns. The pinnas of bats are large and often completely out of proportion to the size of the head. Some of the long-eared bats have ears 1½ in long, almost half the length of the head and body. In front of the ear there is often a well-developed tragus, the equivalent of the small lobe in front of the meatus of our ears. At one time it was thought that the tragus played a part in the bat's sensitive hearing, helping to direct the sound into the ear like the pinnas, but bending it has no effect on the bat's sonar, whereas distorting the pinna makes a bat helpless.

The sensitivity of the inner ear can be measured by investigating the cochlear microphonics. This has been done by Griffin's co-worker Galambos. Cochlear microphonics are produced in our ears in response to sounds of frequencies from 30 cps to 20,000 cps. Bats were also found to be sensitive to sounds down to 30 cps, so their lower threshold is about the same as ours. But Galambos found that they could detect frequencies of up to 90,000 or 100,000 cps. These very high frequencies could only be heard if the sound was very loud and the bats certainly would not be able to detect the faint echoes of this frequency. The sound emitted by flying bats ranges from 10,000 to 100,000 cps depending on the species, but the important sounds for echolocation are usually between 30,000 and 60,000 cps—within the range for which strong cochlear microphonics can be measured in their ears. Two structural changes have been found in the cochleas of bats that might account for their great sensitivity. The part of the cochlea nearest the stapes is unusually large and the basilar membrane at this end of the cochlea, which in all mammals is at its narrowest at this point, is narrower than usual in bats. How these modifications affect hearing is not known but it is significant that it is the end of the cochlea nearest the stapes that responds to sounds of high frequency.

We find it difficult to hear a faint sound just after a very loud one and bats have a greater problem as the faint echo returns only a fraction of a second after the loud pulse is emitted. Deafening is prevented by a muscle in the middle ear contracting to draw the stapes away from the window of the cochlea. The muscle contracts just before the pulse is emitted then relaxes in time to receive the returning echo. We shall see later that the rate at which pulses are emitted rises rapidly as the bat nears its prey. When this happens the muscle attached to the stapes is incapable of contracting and relaxing at each pulse. Instead, it stays contracted so the echoes as well as the emitted pulses have difficulty in reaching the cochlea. This apparently does not matter when the bat is near its prey because the echoes from a nearby object are so much louder and can be transmitted through the desensitised middle ear.

The orientation sounds made by bats can be heard on a bat-detector as a series of clicks rather like the slow putt-putt of an idling tractor. When the bat comes near an insect, the clicks speed up and when it chases the insect the bat-detector roars like a band-saw. These three phases of ultrasonic emission are called the search, approach and terminal phases. The search phase is for orientation and the pulses are emitted at long intervals. When flying about hunting or travelling to and from their hunting grounds bats emit ultrasonics at a fairly slow rate. The vespers emit pulses lasting about 2 milliseconds, and each pulse contains about fifty waves. The number of pulses emitted each second depends on the situation. When flying 40 or 50 ft up, a bat may emit only four or five pulses per second. Nearer the ground the rate increases, perhaps to ten or twenty per second.

When the bat detects an insect and turns towards it in the approach phase the pulse rate speeds up. Finally when the insect is only a few inches away, the length of the pulse shortens and up to 200 per second are emitted, an increase of between ten and twenty times. The high rate of pulse emission presumably enhances the sensitivity of the sonar, so enabling the bat to judge the position of its prey so accurately that it can, for instance, trap a minute fruit fly in its open mouth.

The change in pulse rate as the bat moves from searching to approaching makes it easy to calculate the distance at which a bat detects its prey. By combining bat-detector records with photographs it was found that little brown bats are able to detect fruit flies when they were 20 in, and sometimes as much as 40 in, away. Larger insects such as moths can be located at greater distances and the detection of noises made by the insects themselves, such as the sound of wingbeats, may allow detection long before the bat picks up the echoes from its ultrasonics.

Even without discussing the methods by which bats sort out the echoes they are interested in, such as those coming from possible prey, from the jumble of echoes from other objects as well as from the ultrasonics of other bats (for such a discussion would be unsatisfactory as these methods are not well understood), we can appreciate that the bat's echolocation system is marvellously efficient. It can pick up echoes 2,000 times weaker than the pulses it sends out and it can use these echoes to locate objects with great accuracy. The system, including transmitter, receiver and computer, weighs about $\frac{1}{3}$ oz, compared with the several hundred pounds of a radar set. Although the radar can detect an object hundreds of miles away, that object has to be several yards across. A bat can detect an insect $\frac{1}{3}$ in across, 6 ft away. Compared weight for weight this makes the bat's echolocation system far more efficient than the radar.

The most efficient systems, however, have their weaknesses. As barn owls are outwitted by the super-sensitive hearing of kangaroo rats, so bats are eluded by some of their prey. It has been found that moths and lacewings that are active at night can detect the ultrasonic emissions of bats, with hearing organs similar to those of crickets. This was discovered by recording nerve impulses in immobilised moths when ultrasonics were generated by a microphone or when a bat was allowed to fly around the laboratory. The moth's hearing organs are sensitive to ultrasonics up to 240,000 cps, but are most sensitive to a range from 15,000 to 60,000 cps—the frequencies emitted by bats. No one has, however, yet demonstrated satisfactorily that moths fly away from bats. One multi-flash photograph has been taken showing the track of a moth spiralling away from the path of a bat. The picture was obtained during experiments in which multi-flash photographs were taken of the reactions of moths and lacewings to an artificial source of ultrasonics. The insects' reactions were very varied. If they were near the sound source when it was switched on, they executed a variety of aerobatics, looping and spiralling, or diving at the ground where they would hide in the grass. If farther away, the moths turned and flew away. It seems that when the ultrasonics are very loud the insects cannot tell which direction they come from and so perform manœuvres at random or dive clear, but if the sound is weak enough they can localise it and turn away.

This one photograph is, as yet, the only piece of real evidence that these insects can detect bats in time to avoid them, but it is certain that an insect has an advantage over a bat. The bat can only detect insects when it is near enough to hear the faint echoes, while the insects can hear the loud transmitted pulses over greater distances. An insect is also more agile than a bat and can turn rapidly, thus often being able to dodge out of the way, as I discovered when the bat in my garden tried to catch the butterfly.

More indirect proof that moths react to ultrasonics in a way that suggests they avoid bats was provided by some experiments in controlling insect pests. At the beginning of this century the European maize moth was accidentally imported into the United States, where it is known as the corn borer. Attempts at eradicating it failed and it eventually reached the corn belt of the Midwest where it is now a serious pest. The corn borer or maize moth is a night-flying moth of the type that is known to be sensitive to bat ultrasonics. Accordingly, two Canadian entomologists set up an ultrasonic generator in a field of maize. It was mounted on a turntable and rotated so that the beam of sound swept around the field like the beam from a lighthouse. The speed of rotation was adjusted so that it appeared to any moth like the pulses from a bat. The experiment was considered successful as, when compared with the other fields, the test plot was found to have suffered only half as much damage from corn borers. It therefore seems that this 'artificial bat' must have been scaring the moths away.

The story of the interaction between bats and moths recounted so far is like that of the barn owls and kangaroo rats in that it is one of the development of weapons and counter weapons, but recently the story has been given an unexpected twist. Bats track down moths by ultrasonic echolocation, the moths detect the ultrasonics and take evasive action. Now it has been found that some moths are themselves producing ultrasonics and that these scare bats away.

Some moths were found to make ultrasonic clicks when a bat flew 2 yd or more from them. The bat would then sheer away. A bat could also be made to turn away from other kinds of insects if recorded moth calls were played as they approached them. The clicks are thought to be warnings to the bats that the moths are distasteful and best left alone. It is usual for distasteful insects such as wasps, bees, burnet moths and others to have bright colours which tell potential enemies that they are dangerous. Just as once a bird has incautiously eaten a wasp, it is likely to leave the black and yellow striped hoverfly alone. Warning colours are, however, useless against bats that hunt by hearing in the dark, and these moths have evolved the same sort of defensive equipment as poisonous insects that fly by day, but adapted it for their particular needs.

Insects are not the only food of bats. The fish-eating or bulldog bat lives on the coasts of America from north-west Mexico to northern Argentina and on Trinidad and the islands of the Antilles. Two other species, the fishing bat and the false vampire, also feed on fish, but it is the habits of the fish-eating bat that have been studied in laboratories to ascertain how they manage to locate fish.

At dusk fish-eating bats leave their roosts in clefts in cliffs or in hollow trees and fly up and down over water. Sometimes they can be seen in the lights of a moored ship, cruising low over

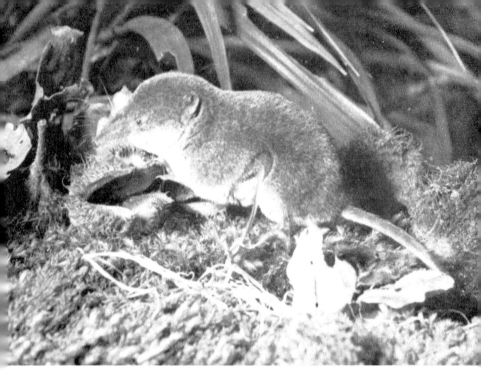

Page 71 (above) *Shrews can detect large objects by sonar and so avoid open spaces where they are vulnerable to predators*; (below) *Mudskippers spend much of their time out of water. Their eyes are set in retractable turrets and are protected from drying up by 'spectacles'*

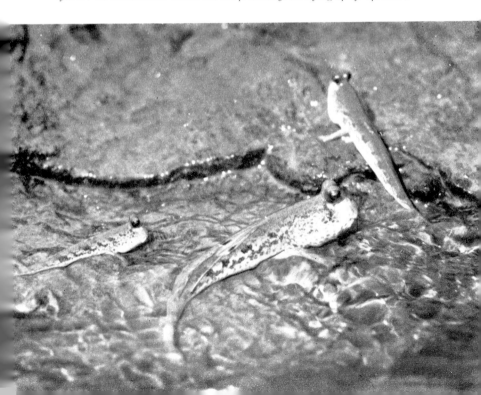

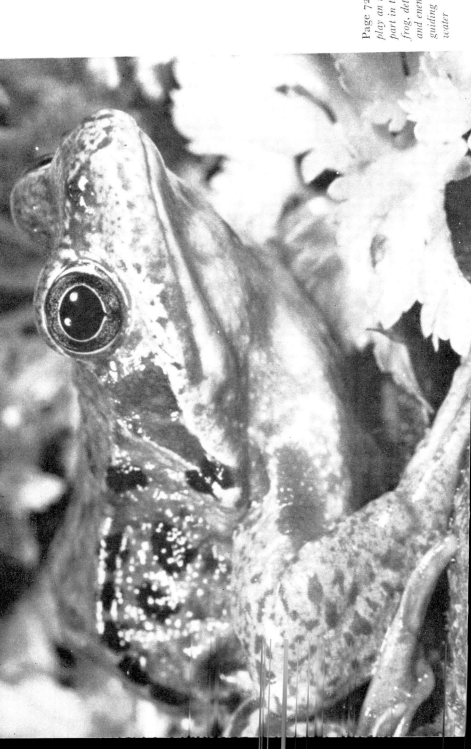

the waves and dipping down occasionally to touch the water. High-speed photography has shown that the bats gaff fish with their long hind claws which they trail in the water. Fish swimming underwater could not have been found by echolocation since ultrasonic pulses would be almost entirely reflected back at the surface of the water. Only o·1 per cent of the sound energy would penetrate. Similarly any sound reflected off the fish would decrease by 99·9 per cent as it left the water, so detection of fish underwater is beyond the capabilities of bats. The suggestion that the bats were dipping their claws in at random seems implausible as even if they struck a shoal of fish this would be a most inefficient way of fishing.

To resolve the problem some fish-eating bats were allowed to catch fish from shallow tanks. They were unable to find fish swimming just below the surface but they would dip down at any ripple. More detailed tests showed that the bats could detect wire of o·2 mm diameter projecting ¼ in out of the water from a distance of 2 ft. So it seems that fish-eating bats catch small fish that occasionally break the surface or cause a ripple. This would explain why fish-eating bats sometimes fish in company with pelicans. They catch the fish as they break the surface while fleeing in panic from the pelicans. Fish-eating bats have also been seen hawking over shoals of fish that are being chased to the surface by predatory fish.

In the thirty years that have elapsed since Griffin took his bats to Professor Pierce, our knowledge of the ultrasonic world of bats has increased overwhelmingly, and at the same time we are finding that other animals are using echolocation. Until submarine warfare led to the invention of devices for listening underwater, it was customary to refer to the 'Silence of the Deep'. Then it was found that hydrophones for detecting submarines were picking up all sorts of strange noises. The reason for the apparent silence was the same as that behind the fish-eating bats' inability to detect fish underwater: the noises cannot penetrate the surface of the water into the air. It is now known that many fish are extremely noisy and whales and seals, too, produce trills and grunts. In fact it is surprising that the sea should have been considered so silent, for sailors had long known that some whales could produce noises. The beluga or white whale was called the sea canary and it is said that the Sirens that tried to lure Ulysses off course were no more than very noisy fish called weakfish or meagre.

The sounds of whales soon became familiar, but not until one submarine stalked a large whale under the impression that it was an enemy submarine. Later it became apparent that they probably also had a sonar system as it was noticed that dolphins and porpoises were able to evade nets in cloudy water. After World War II oceanaria were built in the southern United States and small whales could be kept and studied in comfort. The favourite animal for experiments on sonar is the bottlenosed dolphin. It was found to be sensitive to sounds of over 150,000 cps and to emit sounds of up to 120,000 cps so the possession of a capacity to use ultrasonic echolocation seemed very likely.

The head of dolphins and other whales has developed differently from the general pattern seen in other mammals. The nostrils are on top of the head and the area between the protruding jaws, or beak, and the nostrils is the equivalent of our upper lip. This part is known as the melon. The ears no longer have a meatus, the eardrum being connected to the exterior by a ligament. Furthermore, the ears are not symmetrical. One is placed in front of the other, a condition resembling the flaps on a barn owl's head and presumably serving the same purpose of increasing the ability to locate the direction of sounds.

The behaviour of tame dolphins in oceanaria has shown that they have a sonar system every bit as good as a bat's, if not better. Tests were made by fixing rubber cups over the dolphins' eyes, so temporarily blinding them. The dolphins were able to avoid all manner of obstacles in their tanks, and one dolphin was even able to tell the difference between a water-filled gelatine capsule and a lump of fish of the same size. The dolphins refused, however, to allow their trainers to put a rubber mask over the melon which appears to play an important part in the transmission of ultrasonics. The dolphins were able to detect lumps of fish in front of the melon and above the beak but not below it. Also the ultrasonics picked up by a microphone were much stronger when the melon was pointed directly at it. It seems that this acts as a lens in the same way as the horseshoe bat's noseleaf acts as a reflector, sending the ultrasonics along a narrow beam.

So far we have seen echolocation mechanisms as highly sophisticated systems for catching prey, but several animals have a lowly form used only for navigation or orientation. Throughout the tropics of the Old World live the fruit bats or flying foxes. In some places they are pests because of the damage they do to fruit crops. Most flying foxes navigate by sight and find their food of fruit or nectar by smell. One group, however, the 'dog' bats, uses sonar. In this case it is sonic, in other words the pulses are audible to us. They can be heard as clicks and are made by the tongue.

Two birds also use sonic sonar. These are the cave swiftlets and the oilbird. Cave swiftlets live in caves in south-east Asia and are most widely known for their nests of thick saliva that are used for 'birds-nest soup'. Several species have been found to use echolocation when flying about their caves but, interestingly, the one species that lives in the entrances to caves does not use echolocation. The pulses can be heard as a rapid clicking and are used by the birds to avoid the walls of the caves and to find their nests. They are emitted at a rate of five to ten per second. The rate goes up as the bird nears an obstacle or if the light becomes dimmer, so as with bats it seems that a high pulse rate improves sensitivity. The oilbird is another cave dweller. It lives in South America and Trinidad, feeding by night on fruit. Like the cave swiftlets it uses its sonar only for finding its way about dark caves.

Quite recently another, and rather surprising, animal has been found to use echolocation. For some time it has been known that shrews emit high-pitched squeaks when they explore unfamiliar places or if a strange object is placed in their cage.

This could have been an echolocation system at work but it seemed strange that an earthbound animal that lives in dense vegetation should use echolocation. The manner in which the shrew's echolocation system was established is ingenious. Some shrews were made to run through an obstacle course in search of a reward of food. The main obstacle necessitated a jump from one platform to another. The tests were carried out in the dark and the platforms were scrubbed, so sight and smell could not be used. The shrews were watched with an infra-red snooper-scope, a device developed in World War II to enable snipers to operate at night, and it was seen that they ran on to the first platform and searched around the edges and finally leapt on to the second platform to continue on their way to the reward. If the platforms were less than 7 in apart the shrews would jump. If the distance was greater than this they were at a loss, but until the platforms were more than 9½ in apart the shrews would run to and fro opposite the second platform, indicating that they must have been able to detect it.

Obviously the shrews' sonar is weaker even than that of the birds described but even so it probably plays a useful part in their lives. It will tell them, for instance, where there are fallen logs, clumps of dense vegetation and banks of earth. This is important to small animals that face danger from enemies whenever they cross an open space.

CHAPTER FIVE

Field of vision

Vision is of greatest importance to mankind: Genesis describes the creation of light as the first step in the creation of the Universe; of all the physical handicaps that can befall a man, it is blindness that most cuts him off from the rest of the world; and our dependence on vision is continually emphasised by use of words like 'visualise' or 'see' to convey a process of perception or understanding which is completely unconnected with the use of eyesight. We think in pictures, and cannot immediately understand (visualise!) how an animal's perception works in terms of sounds, like a bat, or smells, like a dog: this is a basic problem in the study of animal senses. So, the problem is overcome by transforming an animal's nervous responses into visible patterns on a strip of paper or on film, or its behaviour is displayed pictorially in the form of graphs and diagrams, so that it can be readily understood, by taking in the information through our eyes.

Compared with other mammals, our dependence on vision is unusual. Most mammals live in an olfactory or scent world, but our sense of smell is almost negligible compared to our eyesight. The reason appears to lie in our history. Our closest relatives, the apes and monkeys, also rely on vision and this is connected with life in the trees. Running along branches and leaping from one to another, with hardly a pause, needs split-second judgment of speed and distance. To fulfil this need the primates, the group of animals to which apes and monkeys belong, have developed sensitive eyesight that tells them instantaneously the exact position of objects about them and how this position is changing as they move.

The most primitive primates are the tree shrews of eastern Asia. They live in trees, have long snouts and a well-developed sense of smell. From animals like these the rest of the primates have developed. The sense of smell has become less important, the snout has shrunk and the eyes, which are now quite large, are in the front of the face. These traits can be seen in other primates such as the lorises, lemurs and bushbabies as well as in the monkeys and apes. The shortening of the snout and the changed eye position enable the primates to see well in front of them, and because the field of view of each eye overlaps they have three-dimensional or stereoscopic vision which enables them to judge distances extremely well. When the immediate ancestors of man left the trees to scavenge and hunt on the plains or along the shores, they retained the keen eyesight of their tree-living forebears. Although man has undergone many stages of development, his eyes still remain the most highly developed of his sense organs and this has been a major factor, shaping and controlling his behaviour ever since.

Throughout the animal world, from the one-celled protozoans that retreat from bright light to migrating birds that navigate by minute changes in the position of sun or stars, the essential processes are the same: light energy is transduced into electrical energy by a chemical reaction within the receptor cells. The accessory structures also have the same basic pattern throughout all animal species. A lens concentrates the light on the receptor cells and a device, in the vertebrate eye the iris, allows light from a limited direction only to fall on the receptors. Sometimes accessory structures are very simple, as in earthworms where light-sensitive cells, called photoreceptors, are scattered over the skin. Each photoreceptor contains a lens-like structure and it is surrounded by cells of the skin that are slightly parted on top leaving a small pinhole gap through which light can pass, from one direction only, to the photoreceptor. The earthworm can do little more than distinguish between light and dark, and perhaps detect movement as a shadow falls first on one photoreceptor then on another. More sophisticated eyes have the photoreceptors concentrated under one lens. The image formed by the lens can be analysed so that the animal can determine shapes.

The eyes of some animals have developed into complex structures. This chapter is limited to a discussion on the vertebrate eye, which provides an example of one such development. The eyes of vertebrates, that is of fishes, amphibians, reptiles, birds and mammals, differ only in detail and the human eye serves as a good 'standard eye'.

The basic structure of the human eye needs little description. The eyeball fits into a hollow in the skull called the orbit and is moved by muscles behind it. The front of the eyeball is protected by eyelids which automatically close if the eyelashes or the eyeball are touched and by a salty liquid which keeps the eye moist and washes away foreign bodies and which sometimes brims over as tears. Light enters by a transparent window, the cornea, and passes through the iris to a lens where it is focused

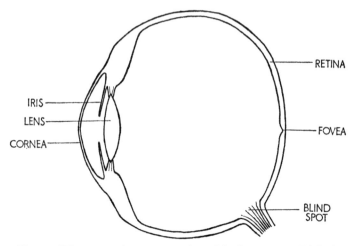

Fig 13   Diagrammatic representation of the human eye. Light is focused on the receptors in the retina as it passes through the cornea and the lens. Focusing is adjusted by changes in shape of the lens. The iris diaphragm controls the amount of light entering the eye. The fovea is the area of maximum sensitivity, and nerves and blood vessels pass through the retina at the blind spot

on to the retina. The iris is a structure like the diaphragm of a camera which limits the amount of light falling on the lens. Essentially, these structures fall into two divisions, the retina with its photoreceptors, cells sensitive to light, and the accessory structures which modify light falling on it.

The accessory structures are formed from the skin tissues of an animal during the course of its development. Their main function is to focus light on to the retina by bending its path. The path of the light is bent as it passes from one transparent medium to another of different density by a process known as refraction. The details of this process and the method by which light from an object is focused to form an image is beyond the scope of this book and belongs more properly to a book on physics. Briefly, light entering the eye is refracted as it passes from the air into the cornea and again as it passes through the lens. A fixed lens can only focus light coming from a fixed distance. In a camera the lens focuses objects at different distances on to the film

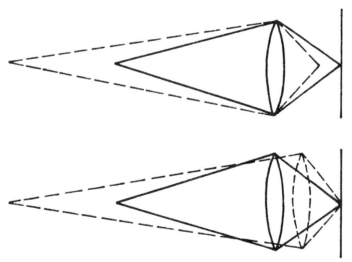

Fig 14   Mechanism of focusing. (above) Only light from a certain distance in front of the lens is focused on to the retina if the lens is fixed. (below) If the lens can be moved light from any point can be focused

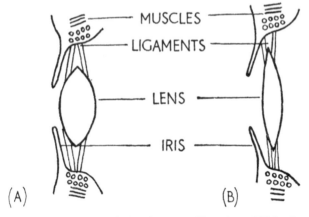

Fig 15   Lens accommodation in man. Focusing of light from different distances is accomplished by varying the strength of the lens. In (A) the lens is relaxed and rounded, focusing nearby objects. In (B) the muscles have drawn the ligaments and the lens is pulled out, focusing on distant objects

behind it by being moved towards or away from the film. A moving lens system like that in a camera is used by some fishes and amphibians. Their almost spherical lens can be pulled towards the retina by the contraction of small muscles and moved away by their relaxation.

More usually, vertebrates focus their eyes by accommodation, that is, by changing the refractive or bending power of the lens. The refractive power of a lens depends on its degree of curvature: the greater the curvature, the stronger the refractive power. The eye lens is flexible so its curvature can vary. In its normal position the lens is flattened by muscles around its edges. If the muscles are relaxed the lens bulges and its refractive power increases. A high refractive power is needed to focus on a nearby object, while the lens is flattened to give it a low bending power to focus distant objects.

Just in front of the lens lies the iris, a ring of opaque muscular tissue. Contraction of these muscles alters the aperture of the ring—the pupil. The most important function of the iris is to cut down the amount of light entering the eye so that the sense cells are not overstimulated. This is particularly important in nocturnal animals, such as cats, which have very sensitive retinas. In the daytime a cat's iris shuts right down leaving only the familiar vertical slit through which light can penetrate. The adjustment of the iris aperture is completely automatic but it takes a few minutes to change from fully open to fully closed, so we are blinded on suddenly walking into bright light. After the pupils have closed down they will slowly open again as the retina itself becomes adjusted to the new lighter conditions.

The retina is an outgrowth of the brain, which accounts for a very odd feature of its construction. In the brain and the rest of the central nervous system the nerve fibres lie on the outside with the nerve cells from which they run forming a central core. Therefore the nerve fibres in the retina lie in front of the photo-receptor cells and light has to pass through them. Not, it would seem, one of nature's best designs; it is almost like loading a camera film back to front. However, sufficient light is able to get past the nerve fibres to the receptors and there is only one real disadvantage. At one point the fibres and blood vessels have to pass through the retina to reach the brain and here there are no receptors. This is called the blindspot, and is just that.

In our retinas there are two kinds of photoreceptors, called rods and cones. They are similar in appearance except that rods are narrower than cones. Distribution of rods and cones over the surface of the retina is not even. Rods are more numerous around the edge of the retina while cones are more common in the middle. In the very centre of the retina there is a small patch, $\frac{1}{2}$ mm in diameter, called the fovea which consists of cones alone. Other animals have different arrangements. Nocturnal animals often have rods only, diurnal species sometimes have cones only and hawks have two foveas in each retina. Thus it would seem that rods and cones have different functions, and this is confirmed by anatomical examination of the retina and by experiments on vision.

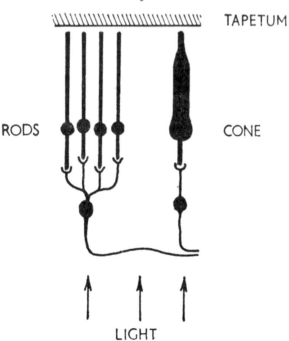

Field of vision

TAPETUM

RODS

CONE

LIGHT

Fig 16   The arrangement of receptors in the retina. Light passes
through the network of fibres to reach the rods and cones. If there
is a tapetum present, stray light is reflected back to the receptors.
Four rods are connected to one nerve fibre; each cone is connected
to an individual fibre

Cones are used for the appreciation of fine detail in bright
light. Each cone is 'wired' to a nerve fibre that transmits its
stimulation to the brain. Where cones are closely packed together the image that falls on the retina will be closely analysed
for each cone stimulated sends a message to the brain. The rods,
however, do not have separate nerve fibres. They are connected
in groups to a common fibre which transmits information from a
large area of the retina. Consequently the image analysed by
rods is not detailed. The arrangement of several, maybe hundreds, of rods connected to one nerve has the advantage of
registering stimulation by weak light. Poor light may not suffi-

ciently stimulate a cone to cause it to send impulses to the brain but the weak stimulation of several rods may be sufficient, together, to fire their common nerve fibre.

Cones, then, are used for sensitive vision, providing the light is good. When we look straight at an object its image is focused directly on to the fovea where there are tightly-packed cones giving a good resolution. Rods are of more use in dim light, hence their prominence in the retinas of nocturnal animals. It is common knowledge that we can see better in dim light out of the corners of our eyes and this is due to the concentration of rods around the edges of the retina.

The ability of the retina to resolve details of the image falling on it, the visual acuity, depends on the density of the photoreceptors, and the ratio of receptors to nerve fibres. An analogy can be drawn with a camera film where the grain of a photograph depends on the density of the photosensitive grains of silver bromide which turn black on exposure to light. In a fine-grain film, the grains are tightly packed so that an image falling on the film is picked out with the minimum of blurring at the edges, and in a coarse-grain film the grains are large and the photograph is blurred. The grains of silver bromide can be compared with the individual photoreceptors in a retina. Tightly-packed cells give a fine grain, high-quality resolution, as in the fovea of our eyes, where there are 125,000 cones per sq mm. The fovea is used particularly for fine work such as reading. Just outside the fovea the number of cells drops to 6,000 per sq mm. Rods are 150,000 per sq mm at their most dense, but because they are linked to common nerves they are effectively 'coarse-grained', giving a blurred image.

Visual acuity is measured by finding out how close together two objects can be brought without appearing as one. This is easily done with humans who can tell the investigator what they see, but conditioning experiments have to be used to test the visual acuity of animals. We can distinguish two points of light which converge on the eye at an angle of 1/60°. It can be deduced that this is the equivalent of two lights falling on two cones that are separated by a third which remains unstimulated. If the lights converge at a smaller angle, two adjacent cones are stimulated and we see only one light.

Of all vertebrate animals, birds are the most dependent on sight and among the birds we find examples of superlative vision. Eagles and other hawks detect their prey while soaring high in the air and owls find their prey under light conditions equivalent to the light produced by a candle over 1,000 ft away. The structure of their retinas reflects this sensitivity. Compared to our 125,000 cones per sq mm, the buzzard has a concentration of about 1 million per sq mm and its visual acuity is probably eight times that of man.

The 'wiring' of the rods and cones can be seen under a microscope but to investigate the mechanism which converts light to nerve impulses, the retina has to be examined ultramicroscopically by the use of electron microscopes, microelectrodes and chemicals. The transducer lies in the spindle-shaped part of the rod or cone that is farthest from the nerve connection (Fig 16). The electron microscope reveals rows of closely packed lamellae or plates within the spindles. These plates contain the visual pigments which alter chemically under the influence of light and somehow stimulate the sense cell to set up an electrical charge. The mechanism of the chemical reaction is known fairly well as the chemicals can be extracted from the sense cells by simple methods or even studied in their natural position. How the chemical reaction then triggers the changes in the cell membrane to set off the electric charge has still to be discovered.

Light falling on the visual pigment can be thought of as a catalyst that supplies energy for a chemical transformation. If a retina is removed from an animal in a dark room and examined under a microscope, the spindles of the rods can be seen to be coloured. On exposure to light the colour quickly fades or bleaches, showing a change in the pigment. When returned to the dark for about twenty minutes the colour reappears. In life, therefore, either the eye must be continually making new pigment to replace the bleached pigment, or the change must be reversible, the pigment returning to its original form in the dark. In fact, it is the latter process which takes place.

The light-sensitive pigment, used in black and white vision, is called rhodopsin or visual purple and is related chemically to vitamin A. The action of light on rhodopsin is to split it into two substances: retinene and opsin. In the dark these are converted back to rhodopsin. Such is the sensitivity of the system that one quantum—the smallest unit of light—is sufficient to break down one molecule of rhodopsin. Of course we cannot perceive one quantum in this way. Many quanta must fall on a photo-receptor before a nerve impulse is triggered and the brain has to receive many impulses before we actually see a light.

We have seen that pigment quickly fades if light falls on the retina, so how does the pigment regenerate? Without our know-ing it, our eyes are continually moving and light never falls on one photoreceptor for more than a moment. In the interval before the eye flicks back to the first position the photoreceptor is able to regenerate its pigment. If our eyes are kept perfectly still with a special clamp, we would rapidly go blind as all the rhodopsin breaks down.

The sensitivity of our eyes depends on the concentration of rhodopsin in the photoreceptors. When they are dark-adapted, and we have 'got used to the dark', there is a high concentration of rhodopsin, and in the condition known as night-blindness there is a permanently low concentration. In World War II when radar was secret, the success of night fighters was attri-buted to the pilots eating carrots. There is more than a grain of truth in this as vitamin A, the close relative of rhodopsin, is itself related to carotene, a substance abundant in carrots. It has also been known for centuries that raw liver, containing vitamin A, is helpful in relieving night blindness.

Returning to the camera analogy, the retina can be thought of as having two films in it, one black and white and the other colour. Colour vision is confined to the cones and in bright light completely overshadows the black and white picture produced by the rods. It is only in the last few years that the pigments concerned with colour vision have been discovered, although as much as a hundred years ago Clerk Maxwell showed that colour vision was trichromatic, or based on a three-colour system. Clerk Maxwell, using the simple device of attaching coloured strips to a spinning top, showed that all the colours that we can see are made up of varying proportions of three primary colours:

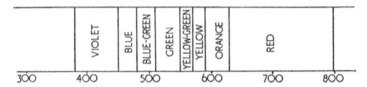

Fig 17 The spectrum of visible light. Scale of wavelengths is measured in millimicrons (millionths of a millimetre)

red, green and blue. Each of these colours consists of light of certain wavelengths and by mixing them in different proportions light of intermediate wavelengths is formed. These appear to us as different colours. Recent investigations of the retina in Britain and America have shown that each cone has one of three pigments absorbing red, green or blue light respectively. Responses to the three colours are partly analysed in the network of nerves in the retina. They are then transmitted to the brain to give us sensations of colours. When one or more pigment is missing from our retinas we are colour blind. If the red pigment is missing, for instance, we are blind to red.

The human eye is a good 'standard' eye. It has both rods and cones and is sensitive to a wide range of colours. It is sensitive to fairly dim light and to movement. We have binocular vision and can focus from about six inches to infinity. Yet many animals have eyes that are far better in some respects, while others have eyes altogether worse than ours. As an animal's behaviour is related to the sensitivity of its sense organs it is quite easy to relate eyesight to behaviour.

A simple correlation can be seen between the proportion of rods to cones and the time of day when the animal is active.

Some animals, like us, have both rods and cones and are active by day and night. Dogs, little owls, elephants and bears are other examples. Strictly diurnal animals, active in good light, usually have many cones in their retinas and in contrast many nocturnal animals, such as bushbabies and rats, have retinas composed purely of rods. Their sight is not very acute but it is effective in very dim light and they can sense the slightest movements. Animals with pure cone retinas, on the other hand, have a very good visual acuity but are restricted to bright light. One species of ground squirrel will not emerge until the morning sun is actually shining down its burrow.

Foveas can, of course, only occur in animals that have cones and not all of these have them. Among mammals, for instance, foveas are found only in man and the other primates. Elsewhere they are found in lizards and fish, but their greatest development is in the eyes of birds. A kestrel hovering 100 ft up can see beetles and other insects in the grass below and has been seen to spot a small butterfly on a tree trunk, at 200 yd distance; whilst the observer watching this needed his powerful binoculars to see the butterfly.

An important structure used in night vision is the tapetum, the mirror that makes cats' eyes shine in the dark. The tapetum is a layer of silvery crystals that acts as a reflector. In a normal eye a considerable amount of light passes through the retina without striking any photoreceptors and is absorbed by the tissue behind. The tapetum reflects light back through the retina so that there is a second chance for absorption by the receptors. Cats' eyes catch 50 per cent more light than ours and they need only one sixth of the light that we need, in which to see. The disadvantage of the tapetum is that it blurs the image as the light is scattered when it is reflected. The tapetum is found in many animals, especially fish. Those that are active by both day and night often also have an iris, similar to that of a cat, that contracts to a slit during the day, to prevent the eye being blinded as bright light passes twice through the retina. An example, less familiar than the cat, of an animal with a slit-like

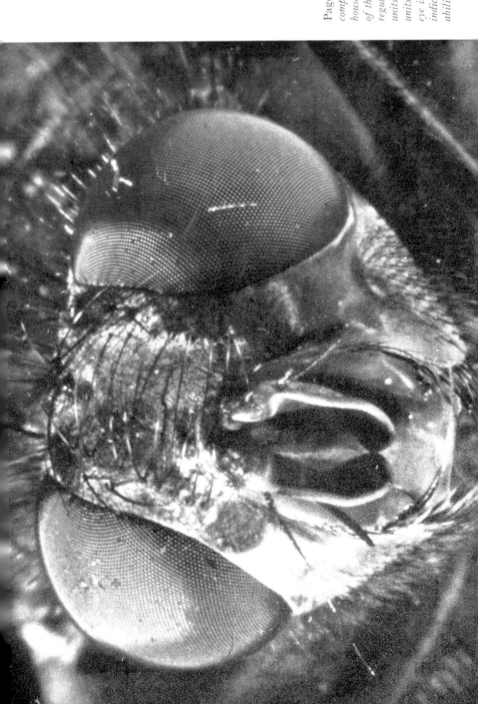

Page 89 The compound eyes of the housefly are made up of thousands of regularly arranged units. The number of units in an insect's eye is a good indication of its ability to see details

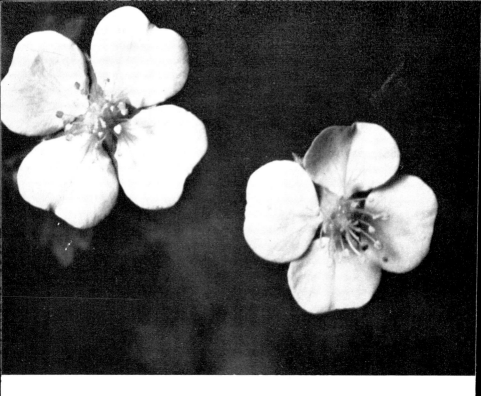

Page 90 *Honeyguides invisible to man:* (above) *Flowers of tormentil photographed by ordinary light;* (below) *the same flowers photographed by ultra-violet light. Insects use honey-guides to find the nectary of the flower*

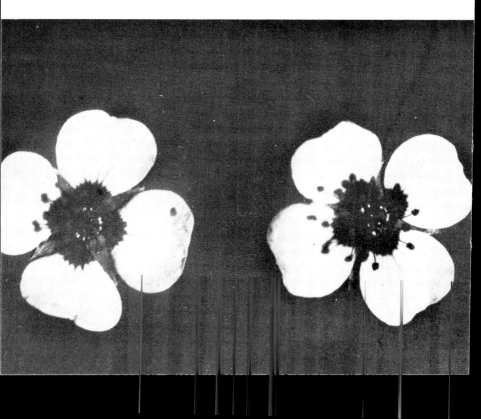

pupil is the basking shark that needs to shield its eyes as it swims near the surface. In some fish blinding is prevented by pigments moving up the photoreceptors from behind the retina, curtaining off the sensitive rods but leaving the less sensitive cones exposed.

Fish and other aquatic animals are faced with special problems of vision. Water absorbs light, so aquatic animals live in a dim world that makes a tapetum very necessary. Light becomes progressively weaker with depth and below about 1,200 ft sunlight completely disappears. In this pitch-black world some deep-sea fishes have dispensed with vision altogether while others have enormous eyes, the rods being elongated and containing large amounts of pigment to increase the chances of catching what little light there is. The rods are also densely packed, up to 25 million per sq mm, to reduce the chance of light getting past them. At great depths the only use of eyes is to detect light emitted by fish and other animals. The light is produced by chemical reactions or by bacteria in special light-emitting organs that are often equipped with reflector and lens.

The functions of the light-emitting organs of deep-sea animals are largely a matter of conjecture. Only with the recent development of deep-sea submersibles, such as Professor Piccard's *Bathyscaphe* has it been possible to see deep-sea animals in their natural surroundings. It is probable, however, that the patterns made by light organs are used to bring the sexes together and no doubt predatory fishes find their prey by looking for their lights. Sometimes the biter is bit. The deep-sea angler fish for example have a lure, like a fishing rod with a luminous worm dangling in front of the mouth. Small fishes, it is thought, are coaxed to within snapping distance by the waving lures.

At the surface, fish and sea birds and mammals have another problem. As light passes from the air into the cornea it is bent considerably and in the eyes of land animals more refraction takes place at the cornea than in the lens. In water, however, there is no refraction at the cornea, and the lenses of aquatic animals are correspondingly more powerful to make up for this.

When they leave the water the cornea immediately becomes refractive and the animal becomes short-sighted. Penguins, for instance, are adept at catching fish underwater but on land they are myopic to an extreme. It is easy to attract a penguin by imitating its call. It replies and waddles over not realising its mistake until a few feet away. Some birds such as dippers and divers have overcome this difficulty with lenses that can adapt from one extreme to the other. From being rounded and powerful to compensate for the lack of refraction by the cornea underwater, they can be flattened out for good vision when in the air.

The eyes of aquatic birds were originally developed for use in air but are now adapted for use underwater. The reverse has happened in some fish that live for part of the time out of water. The mudskipper spends most of its time at the edge of the tide or in small pools on the beach. Its eyes have narrow lenses like those of a land animal. They are set in retractible turrets, which rotate so the mudskipper can see around it. The eyes are prevented from drying up by 'spectacles' of transparent skin over the cornea. Still more peculiar are the four-eyed fishes, one of which lives in the deep-sea and has secondary eyes, complete with cornea, lens and retina, pointing downwards while the ordinary eyes point forwards. The four-eyed fish of South American rivers lives at the surface of the water with half of its goggling eyes protruding. Level with the waterline is a partition running across the cornea. The retina is also divided in two so that light from the air falls on one half and that from water falls on the other. Quite why it has an aerial system separate from an underwater system is not known. It would be reasonable to suppose that it could look for food underwater and for insects falling on the surface, but its usual way of feeding is to dive after its prey then swim up again. Perhaps the upper eyes are periscopes to keep watch for enemies above.

Of all the senses, colour vision is the most difficult to study. In ourselves the discrimination of colour, matching wallpaper with carpets for instance, is often subjective. Moreover, it is possible to be partly colour blind and never know it without being tested. The ability to see colours cannot be deduced in animals merely by finding cones in their retinas as some colour-blind animals have cones which are concerned solely with fine black and white vision. It is necessary to test an animal's behaviour to find whether it will respond to different colours, and here lies a difficulty. Training an animal by conditioning it to perform some action in response to a coloured object does not mean that it is responding to the *colour*, that is the wavelength of the light. It may be responding to the intensity of the light reflected from the object, in other words it may be only able to distinguish shades of grey.

Scientists have, perhaps, been overcautious in agreeing that animals can see colours because of this problem. Most people would now accept that a bull is reacting to the waving of a rag rather than to its red colour, but many are convinced that their pets are able to distinguish colours. One story is told of a dog that had a favourite ball, coloured bright yellow. The ball was lost but from then on the dog, on seeing a dandelion, would excitedly rush over to it, only to be disappointed. Another story, often repeated with different details, is of a calf that becomes attached to the pail from which it is fed. Perhaps the calf may be accustomed to a yellow pail. It will then ignore blue pails filled with food but lick an empty yellow pail. This is a good example of a 'natural' conditioned reflex experiment, but it does not prove that calves can tell yellow from blue. Yellow buckets reflect more intense light than blue buckets so the calves may just be seeing the yellow buckets as a lighter grey.

To prove conclusively that an animal can see colours it is necessary to carry out much more careful conditioning experiments. A German zoologist, Dr Gerti Düecker, carried out a long series of painstaking experiments with a number of animals. They were trained to lift up the lids of boxes to obtain food. They were not only trained to lift lids of different colours but of different shades of grey representing the intensities of light reflected by the various colours. If an animal can really see red, for instance, it will be able to distinguish between lids of red and a grey of similar intensity. The results of these and other tests showed that golden hamsters are colour blind, dogs and cats have a faint colour sense, giraffes can see some colours but confuse green, orange and yellow. Horses, sheep, pigs and squirrels can also see a few colours. Monkeys and apes have good colour vision as do most birds.

There is still some doubt with other animals, one difficulty, inherent in conditioning experiments being that an animal may see some colours but not respond to them. Other colours may be preferred, perhaps because the eye is particularly sensitive to them. Seabirds are known to be particularly sensitive to red. Newly hatched chicks of gulls and their relatives, terns and skuas, peck their parents' bills to stimulate them to regurgitate food. Chicks have been hatched out in incubators and presented with artificial 'bills' of coloured paper. All species pecked red 'bills' more than any other colour. A less precise but amusing variation of this experiment was carried out by Murray Levick in 1910. He placed piles of coloured pebbles at the side of a penguin rookery. The penguins found these a very convenient source of nest material and took the pebbles back to their mates. But no penguin travels farther to collect pebbles than is necessary and takes every opportunity to steal pebbles from its neighbours' nests. As a result the pebbles moved slowly across the penguin colony as they were stolen from one nest and taken to another. Murray Levick noticed that the red ones travelled farthest, suggesting that penguins, like gulls, preferred red.

The preference for red shown by these birds may be due to droplets of oil in the cones. These apparently act as filters, absorbing light of shorter wavelengths such as blue and green, thereby increasing the eye's sensitivity to longer wavelengths such as red, but this is only a by-product of the filters. The main advantage of these filters is probably that they cut down glare from the sea and act as internal sunglasses, allowing the birds to find their food more easily.

By contrast, frogs are known to be particularly sensitive to blue light. The mechanism ensuring this is a beautiful example of a sense organ filtering information from the environment so that the brain is provided with the minimum facts needed for action, instead of being overloaded with superfluous items. The analogy drawn between the eye and a camera can be carried too far. It is useful to compare the lens and iris systems and even to compare the grain of a photographic film with the arrangement of the photoreceptors, but it is wrong to suppose that the fibres of the optic nerve transmit a straightforward picture to the brain. This is patently impossible. There are fewer nerve fibres in the optic nerve than there are photoreceptors in the retina, so there has to be some preliminary sorting out of information. In fact, a considerable amount of analysis takes place in the retina with the result that, on the whole, only important information is sent to the brain. The information is coded into a series of nerve impulses at the retina then 'unscrambled' when it reaches the brain. Experiments using microelectrodes to record impulses arriving at the brain have shown that frogs, although possessing good all-round colour vision, respond specially strongly to blue. When blue light was directed into the frog's eye there was a burst of nerve impulses arriving at the brain. This, of course, did not prove that the frogs made use of the information and it was necessary to demonstrate that they showed a preference for blue in their behaviour. This was done by placing frogs in a box with two windows with screens of different colours placed behind them. The frogs, sometimes assisted by a gentle prod, jumped through the windows and it was only a matter of testing enough frogs with various colour combinations to show that they preferred to jump through blue windows.

One might wonder why a frog, an aquatic animal, should be so sensitive to blue when seabirds have cut down on their blue sensitivity. The window experiment showed that blue light is very good at guiding a frog's jump, whereas green light is ineffective. If we put ourselves in the place of a frog in its natural home among plants bordering lakes or streams, all will appear green except for the water which reflects blue light very well. Even on a cloudy day when a lake appears grey it is still reflect-

ing blue light. Suddenly an enemy appears and the frog jumps
—but where? The obvious place of safety is in the blue water,
to which the frog is automatically guided.

Filtering information like this and the resultant reaction to
only part of the outside world often leads to the conclusion that
an animal is totally lacking in intelligence, but it is only because
the animal is seeing a different world to us that this seems to be
the case. What is obvious to us may be invisible to the animal. A
frog will starve to death when surrounded by freshly-killed insects. To us this is ridiculous as there is little difference between
a moving and stationary insect, but it demonstrates another
neat filtering mechanism in the frog's eye that economises on the
number of nerve fibres needed to transmit important information.

Using microelectrodes to pick up impulses from single nerve
fibres, it has been found that frogs detect four basic kinds of
information from objects that they see. If a screen with a small
black circle in the centre is placed in front of the frog, there will
be no response. But if the circle is moved a barrage of impulses
is picked up from the nerve fibre. Any moving shape will elicit
a response providing that it is small and has a curved edge. In
other words, it has to have roughly the outline of an insect. This
mechanism has been nicknamed the 'bug detector'. Information
from the bug detector is sharpened by an 'edge-detector' consisting of receptors which respond to a sharp boundary of light
and shade in the field of vision.

Two other sets of fibres play a lesser role. One responds to
movement or changes from light to dark. The other responds
when the field of vision becomes darker, as when a shadow falls
across the eye. Together these four sets of fibres transmit to the
brain the important features of the objects in the frog's world.
They detect small moving objects, likely prey, and ignore lifeless
objects but still respond to prey that has stopped moving. They
also inform the frog of enemies approaching and casting a
shadow over them.

The visual needs of a frog are simple; it recognises its food and its enemies and when the latter are detected it can guide its leap to safety, but the rest of the world can pass it by without a flicker of interest. Animals with more complex behaviour must perceive more of the world about them, but even then they will select items of particular interest. The gull chicks pick out the red tip of their parent's bill and when we drive down a crowded street we select important objects such as moving cars and people that may collide with us. Finally there is a philosophical point worth considering. Frogs respond to only a small part of the total environment. We assume that we see everything in ours, but may be excluding part of the world about us and in an egocentric way refusing to admit its possible existence.

CHAPTER SIX

Seeing in a different light

Insects and other arthropods have compound eyes made up of a number of units. Each unit, called an ommatidium, has all the elements of a complete eye and is separated from its neighbours by a layer of opaque pigment. The cornea is formed from a clear section of the hard cuticle, which covers the whole of the insect's body. Under the cornea lies a lens which focuses light on to the cells of the retinula. These are the photoreceptors, seven or eight in number and connected by nerves to the brain. Each one has a rod-like structure, the rhabdomere, running down its inner face. Together the rhabdomeres make up a single structure the rhabdome. The rhabdomeres are light-conducting rods that carry light from the lens down the sides of their retinula cells to stimulate the same kind of photochemical reaction that occurs in human eyes.

Until a few years ago the mechanism of the compound eye seemed quite straightforward, but since it has come under closer scrutiny with the use of microelectrodes, the original theory has been upset. To date, although much has been learned about the workings of parts of the compound eye, the complete story has not emerged. The classical theory was that the ommatidia in a compound eye could be thought of as a bundle of tubes, each with a light-sensitive element, the retinula, at the bottom. Only light more or less parallel to each ommatidium was thought to be admitted and thus each ommatidium would only be sensitive to a small part of the scene in front of it. A picture of the scene was assumed to be built up by the whole assembly of ommatidia in the form of a mosaic of dots of varying intensity depending

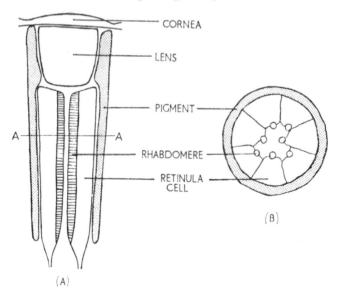

Fig 18 (A) Longitudinal section of an ommatidium or unit of the insect compound eye. Each ommatidium is isolated from its neighbours by layers of pigment. Light is focused by the cornea and lens on to the rhabdomeres which carry it to the light-sensitive pigments in the retinula cells; (B) Transverse section of an ommatidium at A—A showing the arrangement of retinula cells and rhabdomeres

on the amount of light falling on each retinula. The theory neatly explained how insects detect movement. If an object moves across the field of vision it successively stimulates new ommatidia. The mosaic image would, however, be very coarse compared to the image formed in human eyes. In other words it would have very poor visual acuity or resolving power, and this would depend on the number of ommatidia in the eye. Fast-flying dragonflies have up to 28,000 ommatidia in each eye and hunt by sight. They can distinguish movements 40 ft away whereas a worker ant with only a handful of ommatidia can do little more than tell light from dark.

Apparent proof of the mosaic image was obtained by a German scientist, Exner, with a photograph of a window taken through the eye of a firefly by cutting out and mounting it under a microscope. It shows the blurry outline of the window with a very indistinct form behind representing a church tower. Later experiments showed that visual acuity was such that the ability to distinguish two sources of light could be explained in terms of light falling into adjacent ommatidia with light only entering an ommatidium if it was nearly parallel to the tube.

Unfortunately for the classical mosaic theory, these experiments demonstrate the strictly limited use of conditioning experiments for investigating sense organs. By recording nerve impulses with microelectrodes from a single ommatidium it has been found that ommatidia are more complicated than a simple tube. The electrophysiological experiments have shown that each ommatidium is sensitive to light coming from an arc of about 20°–30°, instead of the 2°–3° assumed by the classical theory. At the same time the ommatidium is able to distinguish two lights only $\frac{1}{3}$° apart. According to the classical theory insect eyes can distinguish between lights only when they are 1° or

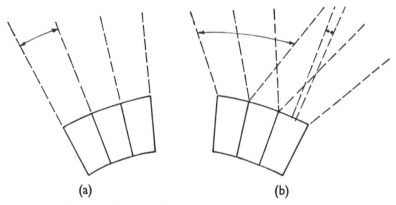

(a)   (b)

Fig 19 Diagram of ommatidia showing the light-collecting capacity as assumed in the classical theory of insect vision (a) and as discovered from electrophysiological experiments (b). In (a) the ommatidia were assumed to catch only light falling parallel with the ommatidia and the visual acuity was thought to be the angle between the axes of neighbouring ommatidia. (b) demonstrates the recent findings that a single ommatidium collects light over a wide angle, and has a greater visual acuity than was thought

more apart, that is when each light stimulates a separate ommatidium. So each ommatidium collects light over a larger area
and the eye has a greater visual acuity than was previously
thought. This means that each ommatidium must be able to
'see' an image and not merely light or dark.

Furthermore, the fields of vision of adjacent, tightly-packed
ommatidia must overlap. The classical theory is, therefore, un-
workable, but a new theory to take its place is only slowly being
pieced together. This is partly due to the time it takes to develop
the new techniques and to digest the vast amount of information
they supply. As each part of the compound eye's mechanism is
explored it reveals new secrets that need fresh techniques for
investigation.

The accessory systems are now more clearly understood. Each
ommatidium collects information from a wide field, and a single
spot of light is received by several ommatidia, so there is a
considerable overlap of information received by neighbouring
ommatidia. This means that a bewildering complexity of information is received by the retinula cells and it must be sorted out
and coded by the network of nerve fibres behind them. It is here
that research will have to be directed to unlock the secrets of
insect vision. The answer may be that there is some mechanism
for sorting out and coding information like there is in the cochlea
of the ear, where the complicated vibrations set up in the organ
of Corti are transformed into a code of nerve impulses.

Meanwhile there is the question of why the conditioning experiments that supported the classical theory gave such low
results for insects' visual acuity. It was thought that an insect
only had the ability to distinguish two light sources if they were
not less than 1°–2° of arc apart, whereas it was later found by
the use of microelectrodes that light sources ten times closer
together could be distinguished. It may be that although the
optical and nervous systems are very good there is a limitation
imposed by the central nervous system. The insects may have
been failing to distinguish close light sources for the same reason
that the frogs, described in the last chapter, did not see dead

flies: they form images on the retina but the frogs are not adapted to react to them. In fact, the habits of some insects show that they have extremely good visual acuity and can discern minute details.

There are a number of wasps that live a solitary life rather than living in a large community like the common wasp. Hunting wasps are solitary wasps that capture and sting their prey, storing it in their nests for their young to feed on. Some hunting wasps catch spiders, stinging them before the spiders can retaliate with their venomous fangs; another kind attacks bees as they return to their hives, but a characteristic of all hunting wasps is that each species attacks only prey of one particular kind. Each has its instinctive preferences for certain spiders, flies, bees, beetles or some other small animal. Therefore, as each attacks only one kind of animal it must be able to recognise its prey.

It is quite easy to watch hunting wasps at work. In Britain there are two species called digger wasps that construct their nests in sandy soil. One, the field digger, finds its prey on cattle dung, while the other, the sand digger, lurks by the flowers of the wild carrot, cow parsley and other plants where flies are so often to be found. Each wasp stalks up to a fly then leaps at it from a distance of 1 in or more. Digger wasps at work have been watched carefully and they have never been seen to attack or bring to their nests anything other than flies. This suggests that they must have remarkably good eyesight, but it is only half the story. Some of the flies to be found on the white flowers of the wild carrot and similar plants are hoverflies that have striped bodies like bees and wasps. It is always thought that these harmless flies benefit by being mistaken for poisonous insects. The digger wasps, however, are not fooled and will capture hoverflies but ignore bees or wasps, showing that their ability to distinguish shapes must be very acute indeed.

This information about the digger wasp confirms the laboratory studies that demonstrated that the insect compound eyes are much more sensitive than had been previously supposed. Unfortunately, it is not yet possible to give a comprehensive description of the eye mechanism. It will probably be some time before sufficient slow and painstaking work has been done to produce a new theory, and it is likely that it will then lack the simplicity of the mosaic theory that made the compound eye such a suitable subject for elementary biology classes.

Not all insects have as good eyesight as digger wasps or dragonflies. Many have eyes consisting of only a few ommatidia and are limited to the perception of light and dark or only simple forms; among these is the caterpillar of the black arches moth. This is a night-flying species found in the south of Britain, living on the leaves of oaks, apples and pines. Sometimes they fall out of the tree, but if they do so they will straightway walk to the trunk and back up to the leaves. One might be tempted to think it clever of a caterpillar to know which way to go, yet if you are standing nearby watching them, they are just as likely to make for your feet and start climbing. They will also climb a stick stuck in the ground. To guide them back to their food the caterpillars have a very simple mechanism, which in the normal course of events is quite adequate. Their eyes are made up of two groups of widely separated ommatidia, called stemmata. There are six on each side and they are clearly unable to form a good image of the surroundings, but they are able to detect vertical edges well. As a caterpillar waves its head from side to side the light/dark edge of a vertical object will pass across the stemmata stimulating them as it moves from one to another. The broader the object, the more it stimulates the caterpillar, so that it crawls to the nearest tree rather than wasting energy crawling to a distant one, and climbs sizeable trees rather than sticks.

Another insect that reacts to a simple shape is the humming-bird hawkmoth which seeks crevices in the autumn and tucks itself away to hibernate. To us a crevice is a complex of three-dimensional perspectives and shades, but to the hawkmoth a crevice is simply a dark object and suitable ones are about 2 in across.

These two examples show how simple, selected features of the insects' world are all that are needed for the control of their behaviour. Like the frog and the 'bug detector', the wealth of detail that is to us a necessity and a delight is unnecessary for insects, and useless, for without filtering out the excess details the simple nervous systems of these animals would be overloaded.

So far we have considered only the appreciation of form in insect vision but it has been known for a long time that some insects can see colour and that they see a range of colours different to ours. Over eighty years ago an experiment showed that insects are sensitive to ultra violet light, to which our eyes are completely insensitive. The experiment was quite simple: ants, of a kind that like to live in the dark, were placed in an arena, at one end of which was a flask filled with carbon disulphide. Carbon disulphide appears as a clear liquid to us but as it absorbs ultra violet light it was opaque to the ants and they collected under the flask. We cannot really understand what it is like to see ultra violet light, but it is perhaps rather like having a very dark purple shade added to everything. This is not the only difference in the colours that insects see. Their world would appear to us as one painted by a completely off-beat artist.

The range of colours seen by insects was demonstrated in a series of classic experiments by von Frisch who is famous for the experiments with 'dancing bees' in which he showed that bees, returning with nectar, informed their hive mates of the direction and distance of the source of the nectar by a figure-of-eight dance on the honeycomb. Von Frisch's experiments on colour vision were also performed with bees. He conditioned them to feed at bowls of sugary water standing on blue paper. Once they were conditioned they would come to blue paper even if there was no sugar water on it. If pieces of grey paper of differing shades were placed around the blue paper the bees still landed on the blue, showing that they were responding to the blue colour and not just to the intensity of light reflected by the paper. By training bees successively to respond to different coloured papers they were found to be able to distinguish six different colours: ultra violet, bluish green, violet, 'bees' purple', yellow and blue. These six are made up of the three primary colours of ultra violet, yellow and blue. Fig 20 shows bees' colour vision diagrammatically comparing it with human colour vision.

The bees' colour range has been pushed towards longer wavelengths than that of man. They see ultra violet but not red. A few insects do see red, notably fireflies and day-flying butterflies such as the tortoiseshell, but to others red is the same as black.

The extent of colour vision in insects can be determined indirectly by conditioning experiments or directly by measuring nerve impulses coming from the retinula cells of the eyes in response to illumination by different colours, so that diagrams like that in Fig 20 can be drawn up. This does not give us a very good picture of what the world looks like to a bee or butterfly. The conditioning experiments, in particular, may give the wrong results. Cabbage-white butterflies choose a place to lay their eggs by drumming with their forelegs on the surface of leaves. When presented with different coloured papers they drum on green or bluish-green, that is the colour of leaves. On

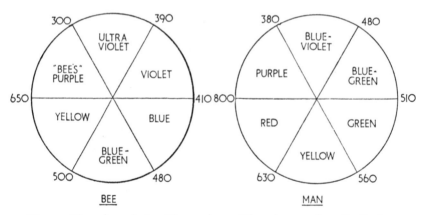

Fig 20　The colour circles of bee and man. The primary colours for the bee are ultra-violet, yellow and blue; for man they are blue-violet, red and green. The colours between are formed by mixing two primaries. The figures are wavelengths in millimicrons. Compared with man, the bee can see colours with shorter wavelengths

the other hand, they feed on flowers and make feeding movements on red, yellow, blue and violet papers but are indifferent to green or any shades of grey. Obviously, conditioning experiments with sugar water would not have given an accurate picture of the colour vision of cabbage-white butterflies.

The colours of flowers are very closely linked with insect colour vision and it is thought that plants evolved colourful and nectar-bearing flowers at the same time as flying insects appeared on earth. Insects are attracted to the nectar and, by successive visits, pollen is transferred from one flower to another. Coloured petals were developed to bring insects to nectar-bearing flowers, although it is true that some insects are attracted by scent and very often it is dully coloured flowers that smell the strongest, if not the sweetest. One has only to compare the green petals of the stinking hellebore with its offensive odour with its odourless but pretty relative, the Christmas Rose.

Before judging whether a flower is colourful or not it is necessary to remember that its colours will appear different to insects, especially if they reflect ultra violet light. Poppies are red to us but bees are colour blind to red; instead, they see poppies as ultra violet. In general, white flowers are bluish-green to bees as they do not reflect ultra violet and those appearing to us as blue or violet may be of several shades to bees, depending on how much ultra violet they reflect.

Some flowers do more than attract insects by their bright colours; they guide the insect to the nectar store at the base of the flower by radiating lines contrasting with the general petal colour, or by a central 'bull's eye'. These are known as honeyguides and act as signposts to the insects. Considering that flower colours are seen differently by insects, it is not surprising to find that some flowers, appearing uniformly coloured to us, should reveal honeyguides when photographed under ultra violet light. Page 90 shows two flowers of tormentil as they appear to us, a uniform yellow; the illustration below this shows the same flowers photographed in ultra violet light with very distinct 'bull's eye' honeyguides in the centre.

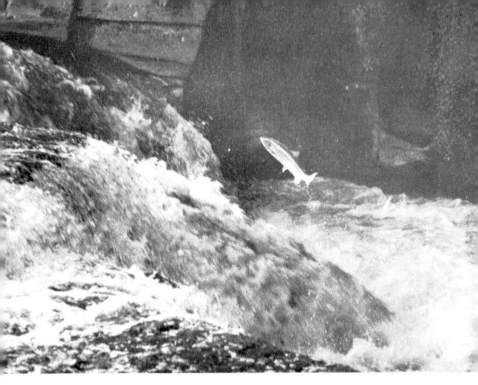

Page 107 (above) *Salmon leaping a weir on the way to its spawning pool. It is guided up from the mouth of the river by the smell of water from the pool*; (below) *Mole holding prey with its forepaws. Note the whiskers on its snout. The whiskers are thought to play an important part in its underground life by detecting vibrations*

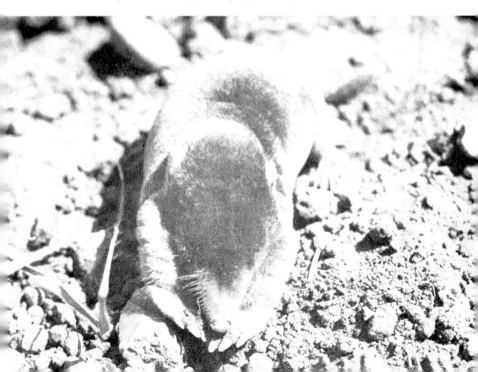

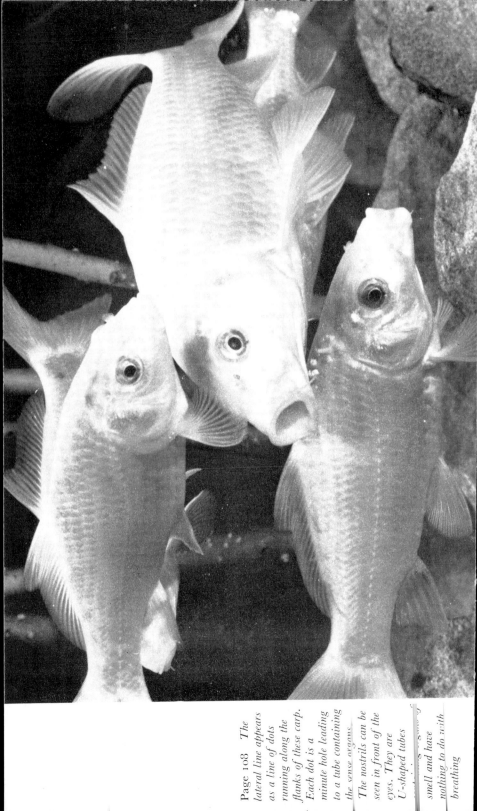

Page 108   *The
lateral line appears
as a line of dots
running along the
flanks of these carp.
Each dot is a
minute hole leading
to a tube containing
the sense organs.*

*The nostrils can be
seen in front of the
eyes. They are
U-shaped tubes
. . . . . g . . . . . g
smell and have
nothing to do with
breathing*

CHAPTER SEVEN

Finding the way home

When man first set out on journeys by sea, as opposed to short fishing trips, he stayed close to the shore. The Vikings first came to England by keeping as close as possible to the North Sea shores and it was only later that they gained the necessary knowledge of the movements of sun and stars to plunge across the Atlantic and colonise Iceland and Greenland. Their journeys were great feats of reasoned navigation but are more than matched by the journeys instinctively undertaken by some animals.

There are two parts to navigation. First there is orientation, or knowing in which direction to travel, but this is of little use unless one knows one's exact position before starting, which is the second essential. Orientation is comparatively simple; mariners first used celestial beacons, and then the compass, to determine their course, but unless they also knew the exact position of their destination, and where they were setting out from, there was no knowing what course to set. It is also essential to check the position of a boat on the journey for the course must be continually readjusted as wind and currents drive the craft off course.

Accurate charting of a boat's position was delayed until the invention of two instruments. The first was the sextant that measures the angle between sun or star and the horizon and the second invention was the chronometer, an accurate clock. With these two instruments a position could be calculated by using tables showing the angles of sun and stars at fixed times. This basic method is still used by navigators whether they are on a tramp steamer or an Apollo spacecraft, and there is now increasing evidence that animals are using the same procedure, whether they be ants finding their way back to the nest or Arctic terns travelling across the world from Ellesmere Island, a mere 1,000 miles from the North Pole, to the Antarctic pack ice.

The ant finding its way back to its nest is not navigating in the true sense but orientating. It has not fixed the position of its nest in space but only with reference to the sun. Having set out from the nest with the sun at right angles and to the left of it, it returns with the sun at the same angle on the right. Pick up the ant and carry it 50 yd to the right and it will set off on its original course and end up 50 yd to the right of its nest. It is blindly following a compass course.

Displacement experiments of this kind have been performed on a number of animals. They shed light on the comparatively simple problem of orientation, but the calculation of position is very much more difficult. It is thought that animal travellers, such as migrating birds that return year after year to the same nesting place, must have the equivalent of sextant, chronometer and tables in their brains. Theories explaining the nature of these mechanisms can only be tentative, as the subject is a hard one to study if only because of the difficulties of tracking animals and watching their behaviour as they travel.

Anyone can watch an ant making its way back to the nest in garden or woodland, but a more convenient animal for experiments is the honeybee. Bees can be trained to come to a source of food which can then be moved about. Their hive can also be moved and in this way the bees' orientation is affected at both ends of the journey. From the simple observations showing that insects steer a course by using a form of sun compass, details of the way this compass works have been elucidated—although the explanation cannot be completed until the mechanism of the insect compound eye is fully understood.

In the last chapter von Frisch's experiments on colour vision were described. They constitute only part of the mammoth study he has made of honeybees' food-finding behaviour. The most important part of the study was that showing the mechanism by which bees find their way home from the flowers where they have been feeding and communicate the knowledge of the direction from which they have come, and the distance they have travelled, to their hive mates. The incredible details of the 'waggle dance', by which this knowledge is communicated, have been recounted many times and will be omitted here as we are more concerned with the individual bee finding its way home than with the way it communicates with its fellows. In brief, however, the returning bee dances in a figure-of-eight on the vertical surface of the comb and the angle made between the figure-of-eight and the vertical gives the bearing of the nectar source in relation to the sun. Early in his observations von Frisch found that the waggle dancers were giving the wrong information and getting lost when the sky was completely overcast, but only a small patch of blue sky was needed for them to find their way correctly. Here was a clue to the properties of the 'sun beacon'. Since direct sunlight was not being used, the information must have been coming from the blue sky, and it was found that the bees were using polarised light to orientate themselves.

So far as is known, no vertebrate animals can see polarised light so here again is an example of animals living in a different world because they are receiving information that is completely lost to us. Polarised light is not a 'kind' of light like ultra violet which we can visualise as being a different colour to the light that we see, but rather a pattern of light waves. Light waves are usually depicted in the same way as the sound waves in Fig 2 (p 24). This is a very simple representation because it shows only one plane of movement, at right angles to the page, whereas light waves vibrate in all planes about the direction they are travelling (Fig 21). Polarisation is the filtering out of all planes of light except one so that the simple diagram, showing light waves in the same way as sound waves are shown, gives a true representation of polarised light. An easy way of visualising

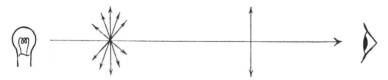

Fig 21   When unpolarised, to the left, light travels in all planes at right angles to its direction of movement (that is vertically in and out of the page). When polarised, the light travels in only one plane (parallel with the page)

polarisation is to imagine oneself standing on the seashore, with waves coming straight in towards the beach. The waves can be thought of as waves of light coming from a source out at sea. They are polarised because they are all travelling in the horizontal plane along the surface of the sea. Unpolarised light would be represented by waves, still coming straight in, but tilted at all angles between vertical and horizontal.

Light can be polarised by being scattered as it passes through layers of fine particles and as sunlight passes through the sky it is scattered by molecules of air. The angle of the plane of polarised light depends on the angle at which the light strikes the particles, so that the plane of the polarisation of light varies from point to point in the sky depending on the angle of each point in relation to the sun. The honeybees see patterns in the sky caused by these different angles of polarisation, and from a small part of the pattern, seen through a break in the clouds perhaps, they can tell where the sun is and set course for home or for a flowerbed.

Somewhere in the bees' eyes is a mechanism sensitive to the plane of polarisation of light. Each rhabdomere may be particularly sensitive to light polarised in one plane and the eight rhabdomeres in an ommatidium may be sensitive to different planes so that a single ommatidium can detect a pattern of polarisation. This, however, is largely speculation and the whole explanation must wait until the electrophysiologists are free to probe deeper into the compound eye and its workings.

Several insects, as well as their relatives, such as water fleas, have now been found to orientate by polarised light. Two Italian scientists investigated the behaviour of sandhoppers— the small shrimplike animals that jump out of rotting seaweed when it is turned over on the beach. When the sand dries out the sandhoppers hop down the shore to moister conditions. Nothing could seem more simple than that the sandhoppers move towards the greater humidity of the sea or even the sight of it, but when sandhoppers were taken from Rimini on the east coast of Italy to Gombo on the west and released on the shore there, they hopped inland. The sandhoppers were not reacting to any information gained from the sea but to a constant beacon. This beacon is the sun and the sandhoppers were found to be orientating by polarised light.

Wherever Rimini sandhoppers are taken they will travel eastwards, the direction that normally would take them down the beach. Elsewhere they may wander inland and die, but nature does not allow for such contingencies as man's experiments. At Rimini the sandhoppers have a simple pattern of behaviour that enables them to survive changing conditions. Sandhoppers at Gombo, Brighton or Miami have similar patterns but their sun compasses are set to deal with their local conditions. Some animals, as we shall see, have similar mechanisms which use other features of their environment as beacons for orientation. Other animals can compensate for being taken off course and find their way home again. This is proper navigation.

A fixed direction for travel is suitable for an animal that has a definite goal that never changes. For the sandhoppers at Rimini the shore never changes and a set course always takes them to safety. But some animals have to find their way to a place of safety that may be in any direction. A set course in relation to an arbitrary beacon like the sun is no use; it is necessary to identify the refuge and steer towards it.

In swampy ground there live small beetles with no common English name but known scientifically as *Stenus*. If they are thrown into the middle of a pool they immediately shoot to the safety of the bank by a most remarkable method of propulsion.

They behave like toy camphor boats. Many insects use surface tension to float. *Stenus* moves by secreting a fluid, similar in action to camphor, which lowers the surface tension behind the beetle and thus it is rapidly drawn forward, skimming over the surface of the pool. The retreat to the bank is not a blind dash in a random direction. The beetle steers for the nearest bank, which it recognises by the contrast between the darkness of the bank and the brightness of the sky. It is possible to fool *Stenus* beetles by hanging a square of black board in the water. They will skim towards it rather than the bank because of the very definite margin of dark and light along the top of the board.

Baby turtles also orientate towards 'brightness' which may come from any direction. Like sandhoppers they are concerned with making their way down the beach. Female turtles lay their eggs in sand well above the high tide mark and the emerging baby turtles have to find their way down the beach. This would seem simple at first sight but, like the sandhoppers, the baby turtles have their problems. From a turtle eye view the sea may be out of sight and the beach may slope upward before descending to the water's edge, yet baby turtles emerge from their nests in the sand and set off unerringly to the sea, by-passing obstacles such as tree trunks if necessary. Haste is essential because there are many enemies waiting for them and if they do not reach water quickly they will dry up and die in the heat of the tropical sun.

Transplanting experiments with baby turtles produced different results from those carried out on the Italian sandhoppers. Wherever they were taken the baby turtles set off down the beach and out to sea, so they could not have been orientating by a fixed beacon like the sun, but by information coming from the sea. Since this was discovered, a number of experiments with baby turtles have been carried out under different conditions. They have been given coloured spectacles and their routes down the beach have been blocked by obstacles. As a result of these experiments it has been discovered that they are steering for the brightest part of the horizon. No matter if the sky is overcast or if there are sand dunes or trees between the nest and the sea, the seaward horizon is much brighter. Moreover, orientation is by a taxis (see p 20): light intensity falling into both eyes is compared and the turtle alters direction until the intensities are balanced and it is heading for the brightest part of the horizon, that is straight down the beach. This explains why baby turtles do not head towards the moon when it is low on the inland horizon. Even a bright moon is only a dim light compared to the general brightness of the open horizon. Occasionally turtles do travel inland. Sometimes there may be a break in a heavy layer of cloud on the inland side and this will delude them. This, in itself, is proof that they are using brightness in the sky as a cue.

Finding the sea is only part of the turtles' journey. Having reached the water they set off to their feeding ground perhaps thousands of miles away. Later they will come back to breed and in the course of their lifetime they will return many times to the same beach. This is true navigation rather than simple orientation because the turtles must know accurately where they are in the extensive feeding grounds before they can set course for the beaches and allowance must be made on the way for currents that carry them off course. It is usually presumed that turtles are navigating by the sun but for the examination of navigation we have to turn to birds whose migrations have been studied extensively.

On two occasions young cuckoos have been brought to me by people who thought that they had been abandoned by their foster parents. Unfortunately it was more likely that the foster parents were away collecting food for the cuckoos, but in the circumstances we had to take the birds in and hand rear them. They were kept in roomy aviaries and were fed from the hand, yet when the time for their migration to Africa arrived they repeatedly threw themselves against the southern wall of the aviary and when released they flew off southwards. They obviously had a powerful urge to migrate and they knew instinctively which way to go. Clever experiments in which the direction of the sun's rays is altered by mirrors show that the sun is the guide. A bird is kept in a circular cage with mirrors over the windows which can be adjusted to make the sun appear to shine from different directions. The bird then changes its position in relation to the apparent 'sun'. Neat proof of orientation by the sun was once found by accident. Dr G. V. T. Matthews, the authority on bird navigation, was carrying out some experiments with mallard. Usually they flew off in a north-westerly direction when released, but this time they were released shortly after the sun had set in the south-west. As they flew off a break appeared in the clouds in the north-west and a red flush showed through. The ducks mistook this for the setting sun and set off towards the north-east instead of the north-west. Such instances must be rare but birds have also been known to be led off course by the red glow over distant cities.

Like the sandhoppers, the mallard regularly set off in a fixed direction no matter where their point of release is. Such simple orientation has a useful part to play in the lives of animals. Sometime during the Antarctic spring, when the land is still snow-covered and the sea frozen to a depth of several feet, small black specks can be seen gliding slowly over the ice. As they approach they begin to take on a definite form. They are penguins returning to their rookeries after a winter's feeding on the fringes of the pack ice. Every year the penguins arrive in parties which converge on their traditional nesting grounds, each penguin returning to the nest it occupied the year before. During the brief summer when the chicks are raised the adult penguins make several trips out to sea to collect food for their offspring, and finally depart to sea for the winter.

Penguins must have well-developed powers of orientation and navigation to find their rookeries, and, compared with mallard, they are easy to study. Being flightless, they can only waddle over the snow and ice at 4–5 mph. Their black backs stand out in contrast to their surroundings and they leave easily followed tracks in the snow. These considerations led John Emlen and Richard Penney to visit the American bases in the Antarctic where they could take penguins from their rookeries and release them on vast expanses of featureless ice and snow. As each penguin was released it peered about then set out across the snow. Its course was plotted at intervals until it finally disappeared over the horizon. Provided the sun was visible the penguin kept to a straight track, but if clouds rolled up the penguin got 'lost' immediately and wandered about erratically. When the clouds cleared it immediately resumed its original course. The significant finding with all the penguins tested was that they headed north-north-east, with respect to a north–south line drawn through their home rookery. (It must be remembered that near the South Pole a north-north-east heading changes as one goes around the Pole because whichever direction one takes from the Pole one is heading due north.) Groups were released at five points in the Antarctic, including the South Pole and out on the pack ice many miles from land. From each place the penguins set off on the same bearing, and this never led back to the rookery.

The reason for this apparently pointless course is the same as that for the observations of captive birds facing the direction in which they would migrate if they had their freedom. The penguins are setting off in the general direction of their winter journey into more northerly waters. In the Antarctic any journey in a northerly direction leads to the sea so the penguins' course is common sense, except for the tendency towards the east, the reason for which is not immediately apparent. However, around the continent of Antarctica the current flows continually in a westerly direction and it is now thought that the easterly movement of the penguins is probably just sufficient to compensate for this current and prevents them from drifting too far from their rookeries during the winter.

The movement out to sea from the rookeries, and presumably a correspondingly southerly movement back, cannot be the whole story of penguin navigation. When out at sea feeding, the penguins probably cover large areas and they must have some method of knowing their exact position so that they can set an exact, rather than a general, course to the rookeries in spring. So, too, must other migratory birds be able to keep to a course and make corrections if the wind blows them off it. Small birds, such as redstarts and pied flycatchers, migrating from Scandinavia to Spain and Portugal sometimes get blown by adverse winds across the North Sea to the east coast of Britain. By tracking them by radar as they set off again and analysing the courses of birds that have been ringed, it has been found that they leave Britain on a south-south-east course that would bring them to their proper destination, rather than continuing on the original south-south-west course and getting lost in the Atlantic.

How birds plot their position is a matter of conjecture. The problems of deciphering the physiological mechanisms analogous to compasses, sextants and charts are overwhelming, but theoretical mechanisms can be predicted on the basis of the observed capabilities of a bird's brain and sense organs. If a theory derived from established knowledge explains the bird's behaviour with no contradiction, there is a good chance that it is correct and that the physiological basis will eventually be found to fit it. This apparently back-to-front procedure has often been applied in many differing branches of science. The existence and position of the planet Neptune for instance was predicted from observations of Uranus and then confirmed by searching the sky with telescopes. The theoretical deductions told the astronomers where to look for the planet. In the same way a theoretical mechanism of position-finding in birds will tell physiologists what to look for in brain and sense organs.

Such a theory has been put forward by Dr Matthews and, although it has been criticised by other ornithologists and will no doubt be amended by Dr Matthews himself as new facts become available, it gives us a good idea of the incredible capabilities of birds' eyes and of the almost uncanny ability of the brain to process information received from them.

Dr Matthews's idea is that birds navigate on migration, or when homing to their roosts, in much the same way as a ship is navigated. In every part of the ocean, the sun is always at its highest and due south at noon. Using the ship's chronometer the navigator finds his longitude by comparing the difference in time between local noon and the noon of a reference point, usually taken as Greenwich. If there is a twelve-hour difference, the ship is half way round the world from Greenwich. The height of the sun at noon also tells the navigator how far to the north or south his ship is from the equator. If the sun is directly overhead the ship is crossing the equator. Thereafter, the angle

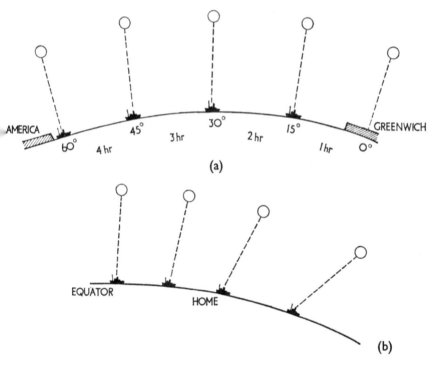

Fig 22 (a) The sun is always overhead at noon and a comparison of the time of local noon with the time of noon at Greenwich gives the numbers of degrees of longitude east or west of the Greenwich meridian. There are 360° of longitude (ie in a full circle around the world) and the earth rotates in 24 hours, so noon is 1 hour later for every 360/24 = 15° movement east or west. (b) The height of the sun above the horizon at noon depends on latitude. At the equator it is always vertical. To navigate, the height of the sun at noon is compared with the height of the sun at noon at 'home'

the sun makes with the horizon declines to north or south, depending in which hemisphere the ship is travelling.

Migrating birds, it is supposed, find latitude by comparing the difference in angle between mid-day sun and horizon at home and the place where they are flying. If they are to the north of home the angle will be less than the home angle and if to the south greater, assuming they are in the northern hemisphere. Both ship's navigator and migrating bird are often unable to see the sun at noon because of clouds but they can calculate the noon position by seeing the sun at another time and extrapolating, by measuring a small part of the sun's arc and then calculating the rest of the arc to discover the noon position.

Another theory of bird navigation suggests that the bird can remember a picture of the sun's complete arc as seen from its home. When it migrates towards home it compares the home arc with sections of the arc seen at the particular place it finds itself and flies in a direction that will bring it to an arc closer in shape to the home arc.

Both theories are based on observations and experiments on migrating and homing birds, but so far no experiments have proved one theory to be more likely than the other. To be worth considering, these suggested methods of navigation should be theoretically within the sensory capabilities of birds. Both theories require that a bird be able to detect movements of the sun and to extrapolate its path. The bird must also be able to recognise noon, have an extremely sensitive time sense and a good memory.

These appear to be within the limits of birds' senses. It is known that pigeons can detect the movement of the sun, which crosses the sky at about the same speed as the hour hand of a watch moves across the dial. Birds can also extrapolate the movement of an object. A falcon, for instance, must be able to calculate the course of its rapidly flying prey within a split second and adjust its own course to meet it. By comparison with a falcon's prey, the sun has a simple movement, travelling at a constant speed on a never-varying course.

Recognition of noon has been demonstrated in house sparrows that have a natural thirteen-hour cycle of activity. When the length of daylight is artificially altered, the middle of their activity period is adjusted to coincide with the artificial 'noon'. An accurate timing sense is demonstrated by birds that sing duets, male and female singing together so precisely that it is impossible to distinguish the two songs. The gonolek, one of the African bush-shrikes, utters the second note of its song 0·425 sec after the first, and this interval never varies by more than 0·004 sec. Proof of good memory lies in the known ability of pigeons to return to their loft after an absence of eight years. So birds are, in theory, quite capable of navigating by the sun; to prove exactly how they do so will be very difficult. It may well be, and no one has proved to the contrary, that they use other forms of navigation. As a ship is steered by gyro or magnetic compass, so birds may be able to keep on course when the sun is obscured by their organs of balance telling them of any changes of direction or even by detecting the earth's magnetic field.

Two hundred years ago Dr Johnson pronounced with full authority that 'swallows certainly sleep all winter. A number of them conglobulate together, by flying round and round, and then all in a heap throw themselves under water, and lie in the bed of a river', and cuckoos were believed to turn into sparrow-hawks during the winter. Nowadays the idea of birds sleeping underwater or changing into another species seems beyond belief, yet their proven ability to navigate over vast distances is hardly less wonderful.

CHAPTER EIGHT

Panorama of smells

The chemical senses have been very much neglected by scientists, perhaps because they play such a small part in our lives and are consequently difficult to study. It is still not even known for certain why a smell smells, yet it is now being found that many animals live in a world dominated by smells.

Smell is the perception of airborne chemicals that are inhaled when we breathe and consequently it is a distance sense. Taste, which is very closely related to smell is, on the other hand, a contact sense, determining the chemical nature of substances in contact with the receptors. But it is a very limited sense, for what we normally think of as the taste of food is in fact mainly smell. Food is often 'tasteless' when we suffer from a cold in the head that blocks the nose, and if the nose is held and chewing forbidden it is very difficult to distinguish between turnip and onion. The tongue, in effect, can detect only four tastes: sweet, sour, salt and bitter. Perhaps a better term to cover the combination of smell and taste is flavour, but these terms are arbitrary, describing our own sensations and cannot properly be applied to animals.

Insects have chemical sense organs in their mouthparts, on their antennae and even on their feet so it is difficult to decide whether one should speak of an insect smelling or tasting its food. In scientific literature the question does not arise. The chemical sense is called chemoreception and the sense organs chemoreceptors. This is a clumsy term, and no one wants to talk about a bluebottle chemoreceiving as it walks over a piece of meat. Bearing in mind that taste is a term properly restricted to the reception of only four sensations, it is best to think of bluebottles and other insects smelling their food.

Smell was probably the first of the senses to develop, as the earliest living things floating in the primordial soup that covered the world must have been able to react to concentrations of certain chemicals, retreating from harmful ones and seeking others that formed their food. Even bacteria have been found to react to chemicals, seeking suitable concentrations of oxygen and sugars, and we now know that the lives of many animals from insects to mammals are governed by the sense of smell. Scent is used in feeding, detecting enemies, recognising mates and offspring, in courtship and in rivalry. There are even suggestions that the nose of man is not so dull as was once thought and that odours affect our emotional behaviour.

The study of smell is beset by difficulties. Because we use our sense of smell so little, we do not have a precise language to describe smells. Terms like 'floral', 'musky', 'musty' are rather vague, conveying different meanings to different people who may in turn also give varying descriptions to a single smell. There is no absolute framework for classifying smells equivalent to the spectrum of wavelengths for colours or frequencies for sounds. To find such a system of classification is the goal of all research into the mechanism of smell, for it is the final proof of any theory that it can be used to make predictions. The aim of a theory of smell is to be able to predict from its other properties what a chemical will smell like.

Several theories have been proposed within the last two decades. Each one fits certain known facts about smell but they all have their drawbacks and more research is necessary to determine whether one of these theories, suitably modified, or a completely new theory will provide the answer. The solution of the problem is not only of importance to physiologists interested in the workings of sense organs. A knowledge of the mechanism of smell is needed to investigate the vital role that it plays in the lives of many animals.

Finding a system of classification of smells and researching into the mechanism of smell have been difficult because until recently we have had no apparatus for recording or measuring smells in any way equivalent to the camera or tape recorder for recording sights and sounds. The apparatus that has been developed to record smells is at present cumbersome and insensitive by comparison even with the human nose. For although a human nose cannot distinguish smells very well, it can detect remarkably minute concentrations of odours, perhaps in the order of millionths of a gram. No apparatus for chemical analysis can match this sensitivity but by collecting large enough samples it is possible to analyse some odours. Body odours have been analysed by placing a person in an airtight cylinder through which clean air is passed. The odours are then collected by bubbling the 'dirty' air through solvents and analysing it chemically. In this way it is possible to tell the differences in the body odours of men and women.

Unlike the eye and ear, there is little in the structure of the nose to provide clues about its mechanism. There are no accessory structures and the receptors and nerve fibres leading from the nose are so fine that they are difficult to study by electrophysiological methods. The chemoreceptors of man and other mammals lie in a cleft in each nostril. During quiet breathing the main flow of air by-passes the cleft except as eddies whirling off the main stream, but when we sniff, air is drawn into the clefts and over $\frac{1}{2}$ sq in of yellowish tissue. Embedded in this tissue are several million chemoreceptors. They are long, thin cells with hairlike cilia forming a web lying on the surface of the tissue that is bathed in mucus. The chemoreceptors are connected to a part of the brain called the olfactory bulb, the size of which is a fair indication of the importance of smell in an animal's life. The olfactory bulb of a dog, for instance, is much larger than that of a man.

We have seen that one of the outstanding problems in finding out how the eye or ear work is the difficulty of analysing the mass of information coming from the receptors in the form of nerve impulses, but the main problem in studying the mecha-

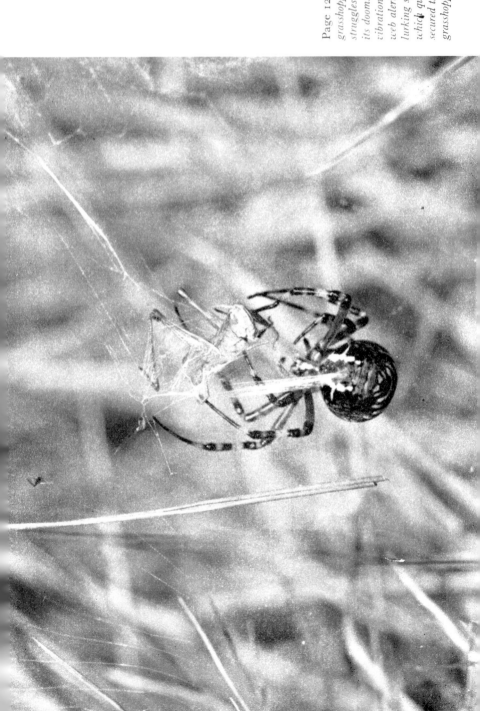

Page 125 The grasshopper's struggles signalled its doom. The vibrations in the web alerted the lurking spider, which quickly secured the grasshopper

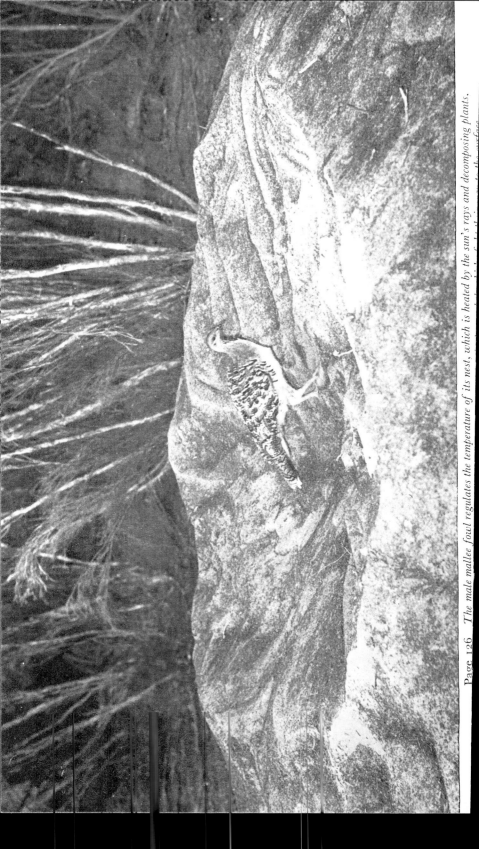

PAGE 126   *The male mallee fowl regulates the temperature of its nest, which is heated by the sun's rays and decomposing plants.*

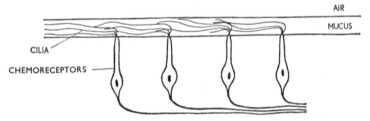

Fig 23   The sensitive cilia of chemoreceptors are bathed in mucus. Scent molecules pass from the air travelling up the nose to the mucus where they stimulate the chemoreceptors

nism of smell is in discovering how the molecules of odour stimulate the receptors. It is true that we do not know how other receptors are stimulated in detail, but we do know that in the eye light breaks down the visual pigments and in the cochlea sound waves distort the hair cells. We have no comparable knowledge of what stimulates chemoreceptors, although there have been many theories. One difficulty is that, as mentioned earlier, we do not know what constitutes a chemical smell, so that studying the mechanism of smell is rather like trying to find out how a piece of a car engine works when we do not know what it is supposed to do or where it fits.

It is easy to go through a day without being conscious of any smells, but if one stops to think about it they are there in profusion. Starting with soap and continuing with coffee, petrol, fish, tobacco smoke, flowers and so on, we find that there are hundreds, if not thousands of smells that we can recognise. The problem that faces any theory on the mechanism of smell is how these smells are related to each other. Many scientists have tried to categorise smells, basing their division on the supposed existence of 'primary smells' in much the same way as colour vision is explained in terms of primary colours. They have suggested that each primary odour stimulates a specific receptor mechanism, in the same way that the three primary colours are absorbed by three different pigments, and that mixtures of the primary odours give rise to different smells. For these theories to work it has been assumed that molecules of each particular

127

odour have some specific character that allows them to stimulate only their respective receptor mechanism. This is visualised as a sort of 'lock and key' mechanism.

This assumption has led to an examination of the molecular structures of substances with a smell to see if there is any common feature in the shape of the molecules that would, for example, distinguish all musky odours from all minty odours. If so, the common shape would be the 'key' to fit the 'lock' on the receptor mechanism. One recent theory, propounded by J. E. Amoore, suggests that there are seven primary smell receptors sensitive to camphoraceous, ethereal, floral, musky, pepperminty, pungent and putrid smells. There is considerable evidence to suggest that substances having one of these smells in common have molecules of similar shape and Amoore suggests that they fit one of seven 'locks' in the chemoreceptors, thereby in some way setting up an electrical charge. The 'locks' are thought to be quite roughly shaped so that a number of similar, but by no means identically shaped molecules or 'keys' would fit them. The study of molecule shapes has led Amoore to suggest that ethereal 'keys' are rod-shaped, musky 'keys' are disc-shaped, camphoraceous 'keys' spherical and so on.

Another theory, propounded by R. H. Wright, suggests that the characteristic peculiar to a smell molecule is its vibration.

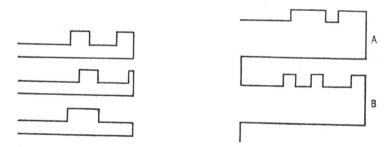

Fig 24 The 'lock and key' theory of smell. The three 'keys' on the left, representing molecules of three odorous substances, will fit into 'lock A' but not 'lock B', so although they have slightly different shapes, they have similar odours

All atoms vibrate and the vibration of a molecule is the resultant of the vibrations of all the atoms in it. Thus every substance will have a unique pattern of vibrations and chemicals with similar vibrations will smell very much the same.

The way to decide between the various theories is to collect information on the shapes and vibration patterns of as many substances that smell as possible and to see whether they fall into a pattern in which similar smelling substances have the same properties.

Meanwhile the chemoreceptors are being investigated to find out about the mechanisms by which smells stimulate them. A very complex mechanism has been revealed. A single chemoreceptor responds to several smells, and the response to each smell is different, so each chemoreceptor may be working in a similar way to an ommatidium in an insect eye. An ommatidium has all the elements of a complete eye and transmits quite detailed information about part of the scene in front of it. Information from all the ommatidia are then combined to give the complete 'picture'. Similarly, a single chemoreceptor may be receptive to parts of a smell falling on it and the combination of a number of chemoreceptors detect the smell which is then analysed in the brain.

The chemoreceptors, especially the contact chemoreceptors, of insects have been studied in greater detail than those of vertebrates, mainly because of their relative simplicity. The chemoreceptors of blowflies are situated in hollow hairs on the feet and on the proboscis—the tubelike mouthparts through which food is sucked. If a blowfly is hungry or thirsty, stimulation of a single hair by a suitable chemical causes the proboscis to extend into the feeding position. It is therefore comparatively easy to find out what stimulates the chemoreceptors by putting drops of various substances on the tip of a hair. Each hair contains between two and five receptors and experiments using the proboscis-extension as an indication of sensitivity or experiments connecting single nerve fibres to an oscilloscope have shown that there are four kinds of receptor. One responds to the bending of the hair, one responds to stimulation by water only, one to certain sugars and the fourth to certain salts. So, if a hungry or thirsty blowfly walks over food or a damp surface, the proboscis is automatically extended and feeding or drinking takes place.

The chemicals to which the chemoreceptors respond vary, according to the needs of the insect. Mature female blowflies which lay their eggs in meat are sensitive to protein. Many parasitic insects are able to smell the host insects in which they lay their eggs. Small chalcid wasps, known only by their scientific name of *Trichogramma*, lay their eggs in the eggs of butterflies and moths. A female *Trichogramma* will not lay her eggs in moth or butterfly eggs that have already been parasitised by other *Trichogramma* females. She cannot see the eggs laid by other wasps and will lay in butterfly or moth eggs that have had a fine hole bored in them to simulate another female's ovipositor, the needle-like organ through which the eggs are laid, but she will not lay in eggs over which another female has walked. She smells an odour left by the other female, so a very simple mechanism prevents too many parasite eggs being laid in one host egg, causing a shortage of food when the larvae hatch out.

At the beginning of the chapter the point was made that it is difficult to distinguish between contact and distance chemoreceptors but the barnacles provide an example where it is difficult to tell whether the sense of smell or touch is being used. Barnacles are crustaceans related to shrimps and crabs and like these animals they have minute free-swimming larvae which eventually turn into the adult form. Anyone who has examined rocks on the seashore will be familiar with dense patches of barnacles and will not be surprised to learn that the larvae prefer to settle near adults of their own species. The antennae of larvae bear discs surrounded by hairs at the tips which are used to search the surface of rocks for suitable settling places. A good settling place is where another barnacle has lain, since if one barnacle has survived to leave a mark it is likely to be a suitable place for other barnacles. The mark left by the previous tenant

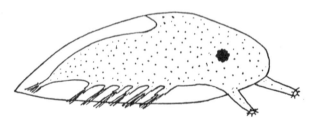

Fig 25   The barnacle larva swims about in its transparent shell searching with its stout antennae for a suitable place to settle. Eventually it fastens itself by its antennae and changes into an adult barnacle, standing on its head and kicking food into its mouth with its legs

is a protein, similar to that found in the hard shells of all crustaceans and the related woodlice, insects and spiders, but barnacles are able to recognise the particular protein of their own species. The unusual feature of this protein is that it does not dissolve in water, so the barnacles are smelling a solid mass instead of particles carried in another medium. It might be that the barnacle larvae are 'feeling' the shapes of the protein molecules. If the receptors in the barnacle's antennae were found to respond only to molecules shaped like these proteins, it would support the 'lock and key' theory of smell.

As well as finding what makes chemicals smell and why they have different smells it is also important to know what concentrations of the chemicals in the air are necessary to calculate olfactory acuity and determine the part it plays in the lives of animals. Olfactory acuity is measured in terms of the minimum concentration of a substance that can be smelled and is usually expressed as the number of molecules per cubic centimetre. It is not very easy to measure this because even if the substance can be mixed in air to give a certain concentration, it is difficult to introduce this concentration into the nose, without dilution. Olfactory acuity varies for different substances. Hydrogen sulphide ('rotten egg' gas) is just as poisonous as hydrogen cyanide, but is much less dangerous because we can smell it in extremely small concentrations.

Man has a surprisingly high olfactory acuity for some smells. In one experiment in which a man walked barefoot across sheets of clean blotting paper laid over a floor, a second person was able to smell on which sheets he had stepped half a minute later. If a man can follow such a scent trail, albeit a very fresh one, it is not surprising that dogs are so good at following trails.

Numerous experiments have been performed to find out just how good dogs are at following scent trails. An early experiment was carried out by G. J. Romanes in 1885. He led a line of twelve men, each one of whom carefully put his feet into the footsteps of the man in front as he walked. After going some distance the party split into two groups and each of these groups went its own way to a hiding place. Romanes's dog was then released and she was able to track down her master with hardly a pause on the way. In other experiments she followed someone else wearing her master's boots but lost the trail when the boots were wrapped in paper. Experiments with identical twins have given an even better indication of a dog's olfactory acuity. When a party containing both twins set off across a field then split up with a twin in each group, the dog followed the twin whose scent it had been given. But if the dog was given the scent of one twin it then followed a trail laid by the other. So it seems that identical twins have very similar scents and the dog can only tell them apart if confronted by both at once.

We are so used to dogs being used as trackers that proof of their keen sense of smell comes as no surprise. One might say that the experiments by Romanes and others were only proving the obvious, but in scientific research this is very often the case. It is impossible to take anything on trust without careful experimental proof for there may be a less obvious reason, that has not been noticed, for an observation. Until one has made sure of the obvious it is not possible to use any fact or theory as a foundation for further work. If this is not done the whole may collapse. Yet it very often happens that assertions are made and continue to be made with no proof. For half a century it has been said that kiwis find their food by smell. This seems to be a reasonable supposition as kiwis feed by probing the soil for earthworms with their long bills and they are the only birds to have their nostrils at the tip of the bill. The sense of smell in birds is, however, very poorly developed so if kiwis search for food by smell they are exceptional.

It was only in December 1968 that proof of the kiwi's ability to find its food by smell was published. In *Nature* for that month Bernice Wenzel describes how kiwis at a bird reserve in New Zealand were able to find food hidden in aluminium tubes sunk into the ground. The kiwis soon learnt to search them for food. Then some were baited with earthworms or artificial food and others with soil. Pieces of nylon sheet were tied tightly over the tubes and more soil put over the top. In the morning the nocturnal kiwis were found to have punctured the tubes containing food but not those containing soil alone.

Compared with kiwis finding their food in the soil, the ability of migratory fish, such as salmon, to find their way upriver to spawn in their native stream or pool is almost magical. In fact, it is not magic but probably orientation by the sun and finally smell that leads them back, although no one has yet found exactly how they find their way. Every year salmon make their way from the feeding grounds in the ocean to the mouths of rivers, then swim up the rivers with incredible determination, leaping again and again at waterfalls in an endeavour to surmount them and reach their spawning grounds.

The salmon's migration is made up of two stages. First it travels from its feeding ground in the sea to the mouth of a river, then it travels up the river to its spawning ground. The journey to the river mouth may be many hundreds of miles, as in the case of Scottish salmon which feed around the coasts of Greenland 2,000 miles distance from Scotland. It is thought that on this stage of the migration the salmon are guided by the sun in much the same way as birds. Captive salmon are confused by an overcast sky and in the laboratory they will orientate by an artificial 'sun'.

Navigation by the sun is probably sufficiently accurate to

guide salmon to within 50 miles or so of their home river. There, another cue is used to guide them upstream. The ability of salmon to find their way up a river to their native spawning ground, taking the correct turn at each fork, has long been of interest to scientists. Salmon tagged before they left the pool where they hatched have been recovered breeding in the same place years later. Sometimes 10,000 or more tagged salmon have been recovered in one study and not one has gone astray. There is now very good evidence to suggest that salmon somehow detect an odour that is unique to their home pool. The chemoreceptors of salmon and their relatives lie in shallow U-shaped tubes just in front of their eyes (page 108). Water enters at one end, passes over the chemoreceptors and out through the other, drawn by the beating of microscopic, whip-like cilia or the flow over the skin caused by the fish's movements. American scientists have shown, by blocking the salmons' 'nostrils' with cotton wool, that they follow scent cues. Salmon so treated were quite unable to find their way except by chance, whereas salmon with their nostrils left unplugged were able to find 'home' even when released in the river at a point upstream from the home tributary. They swam downstream, against the upward flow of other salmon, until they were back on course.

These findings were supported by electrophysiological studies. Some salmon, captured at their spawning places, had water from various parts of the river passed through their nostrils. When water from the actual spawning site was passed over the chemoreceptors considerable nervous activity was recorded in the olfactory bulb at the base of the brain. Water from other spawning sites elicited no reaction at all while there was a weak response from water taken downstream from the salmon's spawning place.

Clearly there must be some odour produced by the home spawning site that differs from the odour of other spawning sites. It has been calculated that only small amounts need flow from the site for the fish to be able to scent it at the mouth of the river. Finding the odour responsible will, however, be a long and expensive task. The small quantities involved make analysis difficult and there are so many possible chemicals that could be involved. The odour may come from water plants or be leached out of the riverbed. Chemical analysis has not revealed any significant difference between water from different streams but by testing fish with water treated in different ways it has been found that the substance in the water which is attractive to fish is an organic compound, that is, it is derived from plant or animal matter.

By contrast, a number of chemicals that attract insects have been identified, although not without a great deal of time and trouble being spent. There has been a considerable stimulus to find such chemicals because they can be used as 'bait' for trapping insect pests. Smell is a very important sense in insects and is used not only to find food but to bring the two sexes together, to recognise nest-mates and organise activity within the nest. In these cases odours are used as signals between individuals and are known as pheromones. Hormones are chemical 'messengers' carrying instructions within the body from one part to another and pheromones are the equivalent of hormones outside the body, carrying messages between individuals. For instance, drones are attracted to a queen honey bee by scent from glands situated on her mouthparts. The scent is very specific, attracting only male honey bees and it is very powerful, attracting them from a distance of several hundred yards. Furthermore the scent not only attracts the drones, it induces them to mate and they will attempt to mate with a piece of blotting paper soaked in secretions from the queen's glands provided that it is suspended at least 15 ft above the ground, at the level at which the queen flies. The queen bee is 'mobbed' by large numbers of drones on her mating flight and during mating her scent is transferred to the drones who are then chased in error by other drones.

One pheromone to be identified is that secreted by the females of the silk moth. It is called 'bombycol' after the scientific name of the silkworm, *Bombyx mori*. Bombycol was discovered by cutting off the scent glands of a third of a million female silk moths. This was a very arduous task and when complete the liquid extracted from the glands had to be analysed by even more painstaking work to find the precise substance that attracted male moths. The method used was to divide the liquid chemically into two parts, so that each contains different chemicals, then present them to male silk moths to see which evokes a reaction and so contains the pheromone. By carrying out test after test the liquid was slowly purified and eventually a smear of oily liquid—4 mgm in all—was left. This was pure bombycol and one millionth of a picogram (1 picogram equals 1 millionth of a gram) was sufficient to excite a male silk moth.

Many insects are now known to use pheromones to attract the male to the female or vice versa, and sometimes one insect can attract others of the opposite sex over distances of several miles. At this range they are unable to tell the direction from which the scent is coming, but by flying upwind and turning in circles whenever the scent is lost they eventually get near enough to detect a slightly increasing concentration of scent that allows them to orientate towards their goal. Pheromones for attracting insects are now found by trial and error rather than by sys-

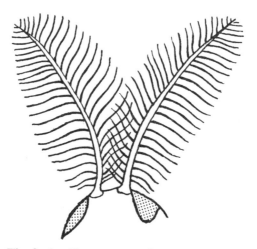

Fig 26 The feather-like antennae of a male moth are covered with chemoreceptors, allowing it to smell a female moth up to 2 miles away

tematic analysis of the raw material extracted from the insects' bodies, because testing the material chemically is so tedious that it is generally quicker and simpler to test the responses of insects to a wide variety of chemicals. It is usually found that they will respond weakly to several chemicals and once these are known it is relatively easy to narrow down the field to find one that is very potent.

Mediterranean fruit flies are a pest of orange and lemon plantations and tests have shown that they are attracted to angelica oil. Unfortunately this is rare and expensive, but further screening produced cheap synthetic chemicals that were extremely good at luring male fruit flies. One advantage of these chemical attractants in pest control is that they are very potent; for instance, one female sawfly, a pest of timber plantations, lured 11,000 males into a trap. Another very important consideration is that each chemical attracts only one species, so that the trap does not kill beneficial or harmless insects, that often suffer more from conventional crop spraying than the pests. If the pests are trapped or killed immediately, the poison in their bodies is not passed to predatory animals who are often killed by eating poisoned prey. Another method of pest control using pheromones is to 'blanket' an area with scent so that the insects' chemoreceptors are so saturated that they become confused and unable to find mates.

Among the social insects pheromones are used to keep the group together and to organise activities within the group. The same scent that attracts drones to the queen bee on her mating flight also controls activities within the nest, preventing the rearing of new queens, for instance. A pheromone, geraniol, is exuded by workers during the waggle dance, supplementing the information given by the dance itself and when a worker stings an intruder it marks the spot with a dab of pheromone and its fellows sting this target so that their poison is concentrated.

Ants and termites spread chemical trails to enable their fellows to find a source of food. Fire ants, which are notorious in America for the pain they inflict on the unwary, lay trails by periodically extending the sting and touching the ground. Any worker meeting the trail immediately follows and so comes upon the source of food. The trail is more than a series of signposts, because the ants only lay a trail on the homeward trip if they have found food. In this way the trail is reinforced only if there is a plentiful supply, and the stronger the trail the more ants follow it. Then, as the supply diminishes, some ants come home unsatisfied, scent is not laid and the trail gradually evaporates. When food finally runs out, the trail vanishes. This is a very neat way of matching the size of a food supply with the labour force needed to carry it home and the operation is carried out with the maximum economy.

Some ants also have a 'fear scent' which they secrete when disturbed, and like the trail scent its use is combined with behaviour that serves the ants extremely well. When the fear scent is released it spreads out within a few seconds, alarming ants within a radius of a few inches. The reaction of the workers is to move in towards the centre of disturbance. If the disturbance ceases, the pheromone fades and the ants quieten down; if not, more pheromone is secreted and more ants are drawn to the trouble. So, small disturbances in the nest are quickly contained and dealt with while large-scale attacks lead to a general mobilisation.

The way the social insects behave has often led people to wonder if they might be highly intelligent. Their complex social organisation, the way they care for their young, gather and store food and defend the nest are, on the face of it, modes of behaviour of animals with considerable powers of reasoning. Yet insects have very small 'brains' which are little more than enlargements of the central nervous system. Complicated nervous activity is clearly impossible and, as we have seen, the trend in insect behaviour is towards simplicity. For instance, the stimulation of one chemoreceptor is all that is necessary to initiate a blowfly's feeding behaviour. In fact, the examples of the behaviour of social insects described in this chapter show that their apparent intelligence is merely the result of blind response to stimuli, but both stimuli and response are beautifully designed for their purpose.

By comparison with our knowledge of the behaviour of social insects and the role that scent plays in it, our study of the social behaviour of mammals is in its very early stages. It is common knowledge that dogs use scent marks, and from the way a dog refuses to by-pass a scent without investigating and, perhaps, adding to it, we can guess that they must be very important. From close observation it is now realised that most mammals live in a world of smells and many of them use scent to convey information to their fellows.

The most important use of scent is to prove ownership. An animal's home naturally becomes permeated by its smell in the daily course of life but the natural smell is often reinforced by scent marks made by urination, defaecation or by the secretions of special glands. Many deer and antelopes have facial glands, that can be seen as pits just in front of the eyes. In October, fallow deer bucks mark out their territories by fraying the bark off the trunks and saplings and scraping the ground with their antlers. Scent is transferred from the facial glands to the trees during fraying by rubbing the face against the wood. It is also transferred by swinging the head through foliage or long grass. Many other animals have glands near the base of the tail. Badgers, for instance, mark their territories by pressing their hindquarters against tree trunks or stones.

It would be tedious to catalogue the types of scent gland possessed by mammals and the methods by which they spread their scent, but in every case the functions are the same: to erect a 'fence' around the territory that will keep out strangers, unless they are of the opposite sex, in which case the scent marks have the reverse effect. The scent also gives an animal confidence and one of the first acts an animal performs when put in a new cage is to mark it thoroughly with its own scent. A male hamster entering the territory of a female spreads his scent as he goes and even marks the female's nest, while other mammals mark their mates with scent as well.

Some mammals have a network of paths rather than a compact territory and the paths of different individuals frequently cross or overlap. Here they place their scent marks informing other animals that pass that way not only of their presence but of their sex, breeding condition and, from the freshness of the scent, their movements. Dogs are familiar examples of animals that mark their home range and investigate the records of passers-by, but tomcats also leave scent signals, although we do not notice them doing so. Hippopotamuses have a unique way of making sure that their scent is well distributed. They wave their tails from side to side as they defaecate, spreading the droppings over a considerable area and covering nearby vegetation up to a convenient nose-height.

Pheromones of mammals are as specific as those of insects. An animal usually ignores the signals of another species, and deer mice use scent to keep species from interbreeding. The American deer mouse is very similar in appearance and habits to the long-tailed field mouse. The fifty-five species inhabit a wide range of country, from swamps to semi-deserts, and in some places several species may live together, but even where this happens they do not interbreed. It has been shown how scent is used to keep the species apart by experiments with special cages divided into three compartments. A Rocky Mountain deer mouse, for instance, was placed in one compartment and a Florida deer mouse in another. When both had imparted their odour to the cages they were removed. Then a third mouse, of one or other of these species, was put in the third compartment and allowed to wander into the other two. By timing the period the mouse spent in each cage it was shown that it preferred to go into the compartment smelling of its own species. This is almost certainly the way in which mice of the same kind are drawn together, even when sharing a habitat with other species. It was also shown that male mice were drawn, in particular, to compartments smelling of receptive females of their own species.

Scent is also very important to social animals. Continuous intermingling and rubbing together give the members of a group a common odour. Sometimes scent is deliberately spread; for instance, male rabbits mark young rabbits in their groups by rubbing secretions from their chin glands over them. The group odour reduces aggressiveness between members and enables them to instantly identify strangers. If a strange rat is put in a pen with an established group it is immediately harried by the others. It is only accepted, if it survives, when it has acquired the group odour. A group odour is also used by honey bees to identify hive mates. Any stranger attempting to enter the hive is killed by the guards.

Recently the group odour has been found to have another function, possibly of great significance. When a colony of rats is kept in a large pen, the population does not increase indefinitely but levels off to a steady number. This is not due to an increased death rate or simply to an increased infant mortality. The population levels off when there are far more rats per square yard than would be found in the wild, and it is the density of rats that is acting as a brake on numbers. When rats, and other animals, become too populous, fighting becomes common and individuals show signs of physical and nervous stresses. Glands in their bodies become deranged and abnormal behaviour occurs. The effect is particularly noticeable in breeding behaviour. Courtship becomes disorganised, females are unable to bear litters and those that do are often unable to care for them properly. In short, the social life breaks down, the birth rate drops and infant mortality rises.

There is good reason to believe that pheromones play an important part in these changes. If a strange male is introduced to a pregnant female rat four days after she has mated, her litter is resorbed into her body. Furthermore the strange male does not even have to come into contact with her. It is only necessary for his scent to be introduced to her cage for her to lose her litter. It is thought that his scent in some way prevents the secretion of a hormone that controls the female's reproductive cycle.

It is dangerous to draw conclusions from a comparison of the behaviour of animals and man, but, nevertheless, it is always very tempting. Overcrowding in human populations is a very serious problem and it appears to lead to the same sort of stresses and derangements from which crowded rats suffer. It is of interest, then, to see whether there is any evidence to suggest the use of pheromones by man. Although we do not use our noses very much we do have a very sensitive sense of smell, and now that we are finding the important part that smell plays in the lives of other mammals, it seems not improbable that humans subconsciously react to the odour of other humans. There is evidence, for instance, that some people can smell 'frightened men' and that this ability is used by witch doctors and others to find criminals. As in a 'country house' thriller, the suspects are brought together and a suitable rigmarole is enacted to upset the guilty party and make him expose himself, because his fear makes him smell. It has also been suggested that we may react to odours of people around us in everyday life, although we do not consciously smell them. If this can be proved, it may be that the use of deodorants has some subtle advantage—or disadvantage—that we do not realise.

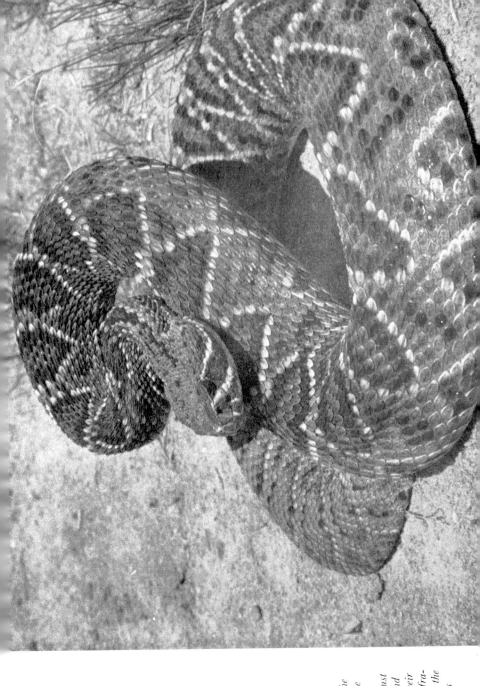

Page 143   *The facial pits of the diamondback rattlesnake lie just below and behind the nostrils. Their sensitivity to infrared rays allows the snake to find its prey at night*

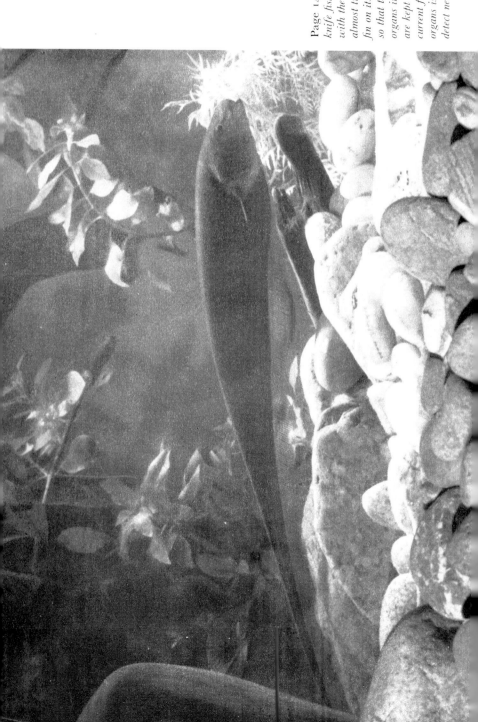

Page 144 The knife fish swims with the long, almost transparent fin on its underside so that the electric organs in the tail are kept rigid. The current from these organs is used to detect nearby objects

CHAPTER NINE

Feeling vibrations

Touch or feeling is the sensation of pressure by receptors similar in structure and function to the Pacinian corpuscle described in Chapter One. These receptors, known as mechanoreceptors, are scattered unequally over the body. The back of the hand has fewer mechanoreceptors and is, consequently, less sensitive than the palm, while the tips of the fingers are packed with mechanoreceptors and are, therefore, extremely sensitive.

The sensitivity of different parts of the skin can be tested quite easily with two pins or stiff bristles. By pressing the two pins against an area of skin it can be found how close together they can be brought before only one pinprick is felt. (It is necessary to blindfold the person on whom the experiment is being tried.) On the back of the hand the two pins can be distinguished when they are 32 mm apart. On the palm they must be 11 mm apart and on the tip of the finger 2 mm. The most sensitive part of the body is the tongue where two pins can be distinguished when 1 mm apart. This is why a mouth ulcer or the gap where a tooth has been taken out seems to be so large.

An important feature of the sense of touch is that although a stimulus stays constant we soon cease to sense it; we feel a hat when it is first put on, then we forget it. The mechanoreceptors on the head have adapted to a new situation. When the hat is removed they are slow to recover and it feels as if the hat is still in place. This does not mean that the mechanoreceptors stop functioning, because at any time we can tell whether we are wearing a hat by consciously thinking about it.

Touch is used to tell us general facts such as what clothes we are wearing and whether we are lying on our backs or sides, but it is also used for special tasks such as performing intricate jobs with the hands. We use our hands as touch organs when examining an object, adding to information obtained by visual inspection. Touch, functioning simply as sensitivity to pressure, plays an important part in the lives of many animals. Creatures as diverse as snakes and dolphins caress each other during courtship, signalling their intentions by touch, while lowly animals react to touch or vibration as a sign of danger. Delicate fan worms living on the sea bed withdraw their tentacles into the safety of their tubes and snails retreat into their shells when molested.

Whiskers are assumed to be organs of touch because they have a network of mechanoreceptors around the roots, yet no one has been able to find out how they are used. A cat has two groups of long whiskers sprouting from each side of the nostrils while others spring from above the eyes and under the chin. Together they make a fan of bristles around the head, and it is reasonable to suppose that they are used to warn the cat of obstacles as it prowls about at night.

In Chapter One it was said that the first step in studying an animal's senses is to find which sense organs are well developed. Conversely, the first step in examining a sense organ is to look closely at the animals that appear to make use of it. Thus, nocturnal, prowling cats have better-developed whiskers than dogs which, in the wild, chase their prey during the day. Gerbils, which live in the deserts of North Africa and Asia, spend the day in burrows coming out at night. These increasingly popular pets measure 4 in from snout to the base of the tail and their whiskers protrude 2 in either side of the head and over 1 in in front of the snout. One can imagine that the whiskers tell the gerbil where the position of the wall of its burrow is and whether there are any obstructions. Aquatic mammals, such as seals and otters, also have well-developed whiskers and these may be useful for feeling prey or obstacles in dim, muddy water.

Circumstantial evidence, therefore, suggests that whiskers are used for feeling objects a short distance away from the animal. It is likely that an animal can learn a considerable amount about an object with its whiskers in the same way that a mechanic can feel the shape of a screwhead with a screwdriver and insert the tip into the groove of the screw without seeing it. Whiskers can be thought of as an extension of the body in the same way as the screwdriver is an extension of the fingers.

Whiskers may also be used for 'distant touch', that is, they may be able to detect objects at a distance from the animal. Movements of an object cause waves to ripple through the air or water and may set up vibrations in the whiskers, in the same way that sound waves make the antennae of mosquitoes vibrate. The vibrations to which whiskers may be sensitive have a very low frequency and are felt rather than heard, like the vibrations felt when a heavy lorry rumbles past. The difference between hearing and feeling vibrations is merely that the ears are sensitive to high-frequency vibrations while waves of low frequency are felt. There is no reason why seals and otters should not be able to detect fish at a short range by vibrations set up by their movements. A whisker will act as a lever so that slight movements are amplified to stimulate the mechanoreceptors clustered around its base.

Another aquatic mammal that may use 'distant touch' is the bottlenosed dolphin. As already described, dolphins and their relatives have a well-developed sonar for locating their prey, so a second sensory system would seem to be superfluous. Bottlenosed and other dolphins are, however, born with a few bristles on the snout. These soon drop off but the pits from which they grow remain. In the adult dolphin each pit bears the stump of a whisker surrounded by receptors. There is no proof, as yet, that these have any function but they could be used to detect low-frequency vibrations or turbulence from rocks or other dolphins which cannot be detected by the ears.

The mole has a fine set of whiskers and it is quite likely that it uses them for feeling its way along the burrows by 'distant touch'. A mole's ability to avoid traps set in its burrow is well known. They block the trap and dig a by-pass round it and it is quite conceivable that this is made possible by their ability to detect obstacles in their path by vibrations. A mole fits its tunnels quite tightly so that it is, in effect, behaving like a piston moving down a cylinder. Its movements set up air currents which may be amplified as they pass down the tunnel and detected by the mole as they bounce back from an obstacle. The movements of other moles would also be easily detected.

The preceding paragraphs reveal a gap in our knowledge of animal senses. Here is a well-known sense organ, the whiskers, which everyone agrees must be involved with touch yet no one has found any evidence to show how it works. The only experiment that appears to have been carried out consisted of cutting the whiskers off some mice. It was found that this did not diminish their chances of survival, but as cutting off their tails would lead to similar results, we are not much enlightened by this experiment. Perhaps the only observation on behaviour involving whiskers is that female fur seals drive away aggressive males by snapping at their whiskers. Seal hunters and scientists have exploited this sensitivity: while moving about a fur seal colony they protect themselves with bamboo poles, tickling the whiskers of any angry seals they meet.

A similarly puzzling organ of touch is the lateral line of fishes and amphibians. Found in most fishes and in aquatic amphibians such as newts, it consists of a line of sense organs running up each side of the body and dividing into branches on the head. The sense organs lie in a tube just under the skin which is connected to the surface by small pores. These can be clearly seen along the flanks of the carp shown on page 126. The sense organs lie between adjacent pores and each one consists of a group of mechanoreceptors buried in the floor of the tube with hairlike processes extending from them into a mound of stiff jelly (page 108). Water flows freely through the tube and any flow of water or vibration past the fish forces water in or out of the pores and along the tube so distorting the jelly and bending the hairs.

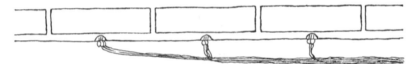

Fig 27   The lateral line organs of fishes and amphibians lie in tubes that are connected to the surface of the skin by small pores. Water flows freely in and out of the tubes and its movements stimulate the dome-like sense organs

The mechanism of the receptors is quite easy to study with microelectrodes as the receptors can be stimulated by pumping water in and out of the pores on each side of a single sense organ. When water pressure is equal on either side of the jelly mound there is a slow but continuous discharge of nerve impulses. If water is pumped in one side, bending the mound, the rate of nerve impulses is raised, but if it bends the other way the rate decreases. Thus fluctuations of water pressure along the sides of the fish are quite simply sensed by the lateral line sense organs and the information passed to the central nervous system.

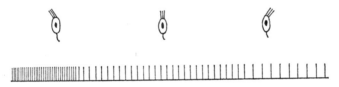

Fig 28   At rest, the receptors in a lateral line organ set off a steady stream of nerve impulses. If the sensory hairs are bent one way the rate of discharge increases, and if bent the other way it decreases

Although these experiments demonstrate that the lateral line is sensitive to changes in water pressure, its function is still largely a matter of speculation. Fish living in flowing water are known to hold themselves steady facing the stream for long periods of time and they might be using their lateral lines to balance their swimming movements against changes in the speed of the current. However, since experiments have shown that they are using their eyes to fix their position relative to landmarks, it is more likely that the lateral line detects variations in the current around the fish such as might be caused by other fish swimming nearby or by turbulence around rocks. Pressure waves which are built up in front of a fish as it swims through the water may be detected after they have bounced off obstacles, in a form of echolocation. Electrophysiological experiments have shown that a burst of nerve impulses is triggered through the nerves leading from the lateral line organs when another fish swims past. This means that fish could find their prey by the vibrations they make, which would be particularly useful for deep-sea fish living in complete darkness. Many deep-sea fish have very well-developed lateral line organs on their heads which would support this idea, but we know so little about their lives that this can be no more than speculation.

Another suggested use of the lateral line is for communication between fish. Many male freshwater fish perform a tail-beating display when courting or threatening rival males. Male cichlids, tropical fishes popular with aquarists, swim side by side in a 'lateral display', jerking their tails at each other but never striking. These could be visual signals enhancing their bright colours but the jerking tails also set up waves in the water that could stimulate the lateral line of the other fish. The effect of tail-jerking on a rival male is to persuade it to retreat but to a female cichlid it is an enticement. The action is the equivalent of a bird's song, performing the dual function of driving away males and attracting females.

Newts have a very similar courtship pattern to cichlids. They emerge from hibernation in the spring and make their way to the ponds where the colours of their skin become brighter. Part of the courtship is visual but the male also induces the female to lay her eggs by nuzzling her flanks and tail-beating, stimulating her both by contact and 'distant touch'.

The function of these organs of touch or vibration is conjectural but the sensitivity of some animals to vibration is beyond doubt. The difficulty of experimenting on the function of whiskers or lateral line organs lies in the fact that it is not easy to show that any of the animals mentioned are using their whiskers or lateral lines to find their way about rather than some other sense such as that of sight or hearing. One animal, however, that is known to be sensitive to 'distant touch' is the arrow worm, a primitive animal living in the sea. Most arrow worms live near the surface of the sea but others are found at great depths or near the shores. They abound in vast numbers and almost any bucketful of sea water will contain arrow worms, although they are very difficult to see. Their tubular bodies, $\frac{3}{4}$–4 in long, are transparent, save for a pair of minute black eyes. They are most easily spotted when they have food inside them, but to be seen properly arrow worms must be taken into the laboratory and coloured with special dyes. The body has three sections: a short head armed with hooklike jaws, a long cylindrical body with two pairs of fins and a short tail with a paddlelike fin.

Arrow worms are one of the main predators on the plankton, the mass of small floating organisms such as diatoms, crustaceans and fish larvae. They float passively in the water then lunge at any small animal that swims past, propelling themselves with rapid flicks of their body. The prey is seized in the jaws and immobilised with a sticky secretion from the mouth. Even herring larvae, larger than the arrow worms themselves, are engulfed. The prey is detected by fine spines around the head which are sensitive to vibration. In an aquarium, arrow worms will strike at a fine vibrating rod held in the water near them. They first bend their bodies towards the source of vibration then strike, seizing it in the jaws, clearly being able to judge direction

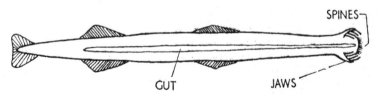

Fig 29 The aptly-named arrow worm detects its prey by their vibrations and seizes them in its jaws

accurately by comparing the vibrations hitting each side of the body. Arrow worms strike at the source of vibrations with a frequency between 9 and 20 cps, but if the source is too close and the vibrations too strong, denoting a large and possibly dangerous animal, they escape in the opposite direction.

Earthworms are also very sensitive to vibration, coming to the surface at night to mate or to search for leaves to eat but withdrawing into their burrows at the slightest tremor. On the other hand their arch-enemy, the mole, sends them panicking to the surface. When a mound of earth erupts on the ground, a sure sign that a mole is hunting underneath, there is a good chance of seeing worms come tumbling out, almost springing into the air in frantic attempts to escape. One or two will suddenly be drawn back in but the lucky ones continue their flight across the ground for 10 ft or more without slackening speed. The same reaction can be obtained by pushing a stick into the ground and wriggling it, but this is apparently a poor imitation of a mole digging because the worms that come to the surface do not show the same panic that a mole evokes.

Whirligig beetles live on the surface of ponds where large numbers can be seen rushing madly about, but never colliding with each other. The antennae of each whirligig rests lightly on the surface of the water and vibrations passing through the water stimulate mechanoreceptors at the base of the antennae. By comparing the stimulation of each antenna a whirligig can detect the movements of its fellows as well as the struggles of other insects trapped in the water on which it feeds.

Spiders have the help of a web to detect the presence of their prey through vibrations. The web has two functions. It holds the prey until the spider can grapple with it, but primarily it is an extension of the spider's body, stimulating vibration sense organs at the base of each leg. Whilst tucked away in its hiding place, the spider can pick up the low-frequency vibrations set up by the struggling prey. The most familiar web is the orb web of the garden spider that shows up so well in the undergrowth after the morning's dew. Sometimes the spider can be seen sitting in the middle of the web but more often it is lurking under a leaf on the edge of the web. Equally familiar is the cobweb of the house spider, which is in the form of a tray suspended in a corner or crevice. In one part of the tray there is a silk tube leading down into the crevice. Here the spider waits to rush out and capture any fly that blunders into its web.

The behaviour of a garden spider can be watched by rapidly vibrating a grass stem in a corner of the web. The spider comes rushing out to the centre of the web, turns to face the source of vibration and runs towards it, only to find that it has been fooled. Having been brought out by vibration it finally identifies its prey by sight and smell, for inanimate objects are cut out of the web and dropped. Spiders do not chase all sources of vibration but only those within a certain range of frequencies.

Over fifty years ago an American naturalist, W. M. Barrows, studied the behaviour of orb web spiders living in the porch of his house. He made an adjustable vibrator by attaching a fine bristle to the clapper of an electric bell and used it to find the spiders' behaviour towards vibrations of different frequencies. Large spiders reacted to vibrations with frequencies between 24 and 300 cps, covering the wingbeat frequencies of insects such as house flies. Smaller spiders were found to be sensitive to higher frequencies, between 100 and 500 cps, that is to the faster wingbeats of smaller insects. Another American studied the house spiders on the campus of his university. He could entice them out of their hiding places with vibrations of between 400 and 700 cps. Higher frequencies, however, alarmed the spiders and they ran back to shelter or even jumped to the ground. Why high frequencies, and even handclaps, should frighten spiders was not explained. Presumably such vibrations signal danger but it is hard to think of an enemy that emits such vibrations.

CHAPTER TEN

Heat, cold and comfort

The sense of temperature is different from other senses in several ways. We are only conscious of extremes in temperature when we feel hot or cold, but nevertheless are responding to temperature all the time. The amount of heat gained from or lost to our surroundings is continually being balanced against heat produced by body activities such as exercise, shivering or sweating, and our body temperature is kept constant at 98·4° F. If our temperature rises through fever or exertion we sweat, covering the skin with a layer of fluid which, by evaporating, cools us, or, if our temperature falls, due to sitting in a draught for instance, we shiver, our muscles contracting and relaxing rapidly to produce heat.

Animals that regulate their body temperatures within fine limits, by physiological means, are termed 'warm-blooded'. Only mammals and birds are warm-blooded. All other animals are cold-blooded, the body temperature being dependent on the temperature of the environment. Warm-blooded and cold-blooded are not very good terms because a hibernating mammal has quite cool blood while a tropical insect or reptile may have comparatively warm blood, and for this reason the terms homoithermous and poikilothermous are preferred. Even so, observations showing that the temperature of poikilothermous animals rose and fell with that of the environment were made in the laboratory on captive animals. Their natural behaviour was overlooked, and some poikilothermous animals can control their body temperatures quite considerably in their natural state.

It is a constant body temperature that makes the temperature sense different from others. Other sense organs have a zero point at which they are receiving no energy from the environment, and from zero they respond increasingly as more and more energy falls on them. When there is no light we see nothing, then as light gets stronger, as at the break of day, we see an increasingly bright light. The same is true of sound; we hear nothing or sounds of different volume. Temperature is different, for there is always heat about us and instead of measuring temperature from a zero point it is compared with the normal body temperature. As a result we talk of two kinds of temperature sensation: anything lower than normal is cold or cool, anything higher is hot or warm. Cold and hot are relative terms: if a hand has been in iced water, water from the cold tap seems warm; but this same cold water will feel cold, if the hand has been in contact with hot water.

These facts have not made the study of temperature sense easy. Consider the following simple experiments. Place one finger in hot water and another in cold water, then place them in tepid water. The first finger will feel cold and the second hot. After a while, as they become used to this new temperature, both will feel neither cold nor hot. From this we may conclude that temperature sense organs are responding to a rate of change from hot to cold, or vice versa, rather than to an absolute level of stimulation as do the ears or eyes. When the sense organs have become adapted to a certain temperature it becomes a new 'zero point' from which further changes are measured. There is, however, a complication. Press a cold object against your skin, then remove it. The feeling of coldness will persist for some time even though the skin must be warming up again. As yet this has not been explained.

It is really inaccurate to talk of temperature sense *organs* as generally temperature is sensed by simple receptors embedded in tissue with no accessory structures. They are consequently difficult to locate and study, but some electrophysiological work has shown that there are two kinds of temperature receptor: hot receptors and cold receptors, which helps to explain some of the strange observations on temperature sensation just described. Neither of these receptors triggers nerve impulses in a simple increasing relation to the strength of stimulus, as happens in the ear for example. Their response is related to the rate of change in temperature and at a fixed temperature the nervous response of a receptor remains steady.

How impulses from these receptors, and probably others, combine to give us the familiar sensation of temperature is not known, but even if the physiological basis of temperature sensation is not properly understood there is no drawback to discussing the effect of temperature on the lives of ourselves and other animals. Once again, temperature sensation is different from other senses. With the exception of a few animals, such as the mallee fowl, bugs and snakes described at the end of this chapter, the temperature sense is concerned with an animal's well-being and comfort rather than with orientation or the location of food, enemies and mates. It is mainly an inward-looking sense, examining the environment inside the animal rather than its surroundings. The aim is nearly always to keep the animal's body at a constant and optimum temperature either by internal activities, such as sweating or shivering or by external activities, such as seeking the shade or basking.

The care with which our body temperature is kept constant is an indication of the importance of a level temperature for the correct working of the body. It is not for nothing that having one's temperature taken is the first step in diagnosis and that a slight 'temperature' is an unhealthy sign, yet it has been found that the temperature of mouth or skin is not directly related to whether we sweat or shiver. The temperature of the inside of the body is the important factor. The actual site of temperature regulation is at the base of the brain, in the hypothalamus which acts as a thermostat, like that in a domestic hot water system. If the blood passing through the hypothalamus is too hot, the hypothalamus sets in motion a lowering of the blood temperature: the blood vessels of the skin dilate so that extra blood flows through them carrying heat from deep inside the body and sweating allows this heat to be lost from the skin to the surrounding air by evaporation. When the blood has cooled again, these activities cease.

These mechanisms are not sufficient to keep temperature constant when the environment becomes extremely hot or cold. It is therefore necessary to take further action before the temperature regulating mechanism breaks down, and even at less extreme temperatures further action can save energy being lost through shivering or water being lost through sweating. Human beings can change clothes to adjust the amount of insulation around their bodies, or move to more comfortable surroundings, and within their limitations animals do the same sort of things.

The domestic cat, for instance, is the symbol of comfort. It may not spend any more time resting or sleeping than a dog but it always seems more relaxed and comfortable. A German scientist once investigated the sleeping postures of his cat, relating them to the air temperature and the place where the cat had chosen to sleep. Some of his observations were, inevitably, obvious. The cat preferred warm places and chose to sleep in front of a fire or to lie on heat-retaining cushions rather than on bare flagstones, but the scientist's 392 observations also showed that the cat's sleeping posture depended on the temperature of the surrounding air. At the lowest temperatures the cat curled up into what was called the full circle. This hardly needs describing; the cat curled round so that its head and paws were tucked up together against the belly with the tail wrapped round them. As the temperature rose the cat uncurled a little to the three-quarter circle, then the half circle and was finally lying fully stretched out. Surprisingly, slightly warmer conditions made it curl a little into the flat curve but why this should be so was not explained.

A cat changing its position as it sleeps in a warm room is almost indulging in luxury, but to some other animals the temperature of the air around them, as it varies considerably, is a very important factor in their lives. Many animals go to sleep for long periods when conditions are bad, slowing down or suspending their body processes. Sleep is not strictly the correct term, although many of the characteristics are the same as ordinary sleep; for instance, the breathing and pulse rates slow down. The thermostat in the hypothalamus is 'turned down' so that the body temperature drops to a low level and body processes, like digestion, slow down. In this state the animal can survive without feeding for long periods.

In hot countries food may be short in the hot season when the vegetation withers and many animals go into aestivation or summer sleep. Farther north, winter is the time of shortage and animals hibernate. Strictly speaking hibernation should mean winter sleep only, but it has come to mean any form of prolonged sleep. In recent years we have learned a great deal about the mechanism of hibernation; what conditions initiate it and how the animal survives a low body temperature. The more the subject has been investigated, the more complicated hibernation has proved to be. It used to be thought that hibernating animals went to sleep in the autumn and never awoke until spring, but it has now been found that in mild weather they often wake up for a few days and go out looking for food. Even dormice, portrayed by Lewis Carroll as the sleepiest of animals, wake up in winter for a quick meal, and bats come out in mild weather to feed on insects that also become active.

The main point of hibernation is, however, to allow the animal to survive a lean period. Some small animals, like mice and squirrels, survive the winter by making caches of food, but hibernating animals store food in their bodies as fat. As the body temperature is low and the body processes are slowed down, the fat is used up very slowly. During hibernation the body temperature must remain steady and not fall too low. When the temperature of a hibernating animal does fall it has to burn extra food to keep its body just warm enough to survive. It is now realised that animals hibernating snugly in their nests are not completely cut off and safe from the outside world. Many of them do not survive the winter because they drain their reserves too quickly trying to keep warm.

For hundreds of years scientists have known that some animals have a layer of fat that is brown instead of white and as it was found to be present in many animals that hibernate, it was called the hibernating gland although no one knew its function. Then newborn animals were also found to have brown fat, including human babies with a layer of brown fat between the shoulder blades, down the spine and around the neck. It was discovered that cells in brown fat tissue have many more fat droplets than those in white fat and they can 'burn' this fat to provide heat much more rapidly than the white. So when the blood temperature goes down, the hypothalamus sends signals to the brown fat tissue which produces heat that is carried round the body by the blood. Babies and other new-born animals cannot shiver to keep warm, and their brown fat acts as a built-in hot water bottle.

Most animals lose their brown fat when they grow up but some keep it all their lives. It used to be a mystery how house mice could survive in cold stores but it is now known that they retain and make use of brown fat throughout their lives, as do hibernating animals. As the temperature drops in winter the brown fat warms up the animal, keeping its body temperature constant. Then in spring the thermostat is 'turned up', large quantities of fat are burnt in a short time and the animal quickly returns to its normal temperature and wakes up.

Despite the life-saving properties of brown fat, animals must still guard against the temperature of their surroundings falling too low. Some animals, like the hedgehog, are protected by the insulation of their nests but others, like bats, wake up if the temperature falls too low and seek a warmer place to sleep. Horseshoe bats live in caves and throughout the winter they move about their cave or even fly from one cave to another in search of a roof where the temperature is reasonably high, from which to hang, and they may sometimes huddle together to conserve heat as well.

The behaviour of the cat and the bats in response to temperature changes is rather different to the examples of animal behaviour discussed already in connection with other senses. Here, they are not reacting to the outside world like a kangaroo rat avoiding an owl or a frog leaping towards water. Their behaviour shows examples of reaction to their internal environment which they then try to regulate.

Poikilothermous animals are able to regulate their body temperature to some extent by their behaviour. Simply, this means coming out into the sun to warm up and retiring to the shade when too hot, but some desert-living reptiles have quite an elaborate timetable for avoiding the extremes of temperature from the cold of the desert night to the intense heat of the midday sun. This is a good example of the interaction between an

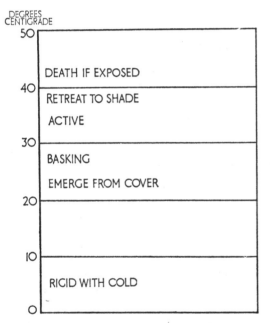

Fig 30 The activities of a desert lizard in relation to temperature. At night the temperature drops and the lizard may become rigid with cold. As the sun rises, the lizard's body warms and it emerges to bask. When it is fully warmed it becomes active and feeds, retreating to shade when the sun becomes too hot. In the second half of the day the procedure is reversed

animal and its environment in order to bring the greatest benefit to the animal. Desert lizards spend the night lying up in crevices, under rocks or buried in the sand. When the sun comes up and starts to warm the ground the lizards, which will be almost rigid with cold, slowly thaw out and crawl into the sun to bask, turning their bodies broadside to the sun's rays so that they present the maximum area for absorbing heat. The body temperature rises until it is about the same as that of active homoithermous animals, roughly 99°–100° F, and the lizards are then ready for the day's activities, searching for food or a mate and defending their territories. As the sun rises higher the rocks and sand become hot and the lizards lift their bodies off the ground so that they do not overheat, then, as mid-day approaches they retire to shelter under rocks or in the shade of scanty desert plants. Later they emerge again and when not active face the sun so that only a small area is presented for absorption of heat. Body temperature is kept high at the end of the day by hugging the ground which holds its heat longer than the air, and by keeping active. Eventually, however, the lizards have to retire to their refuges, safe from enemies which they cannot escape and from losing their heat by radiation.

The lizard's method of temperature regulation is satisfactory as far as it goes, but without the homoithermous animals' ability to keep warm by generating heat within the body, reptiles and other poikilothermous animals are severely limited as to the places where they can live. The reason why large reptiles are so rarely found outside the tropics is that in a cold climate they would take such a long time to warm up each morning that quite often they would never warm up at all, and perish.

For the same reason large insects are not found in the cooler parts of the world. Their methods of temperature control are very similar to those of reptiles. They shelter from extremes of heat and cold and bask in the sun before taking off. Some can, however, raise their body temperatures by muscular activity such as fluttering their wings. Some moths are said to be unable to fly until the body temperature has been raised to 90°–96° F, the equivalent to an athlete doing warming-up exercises. Ground beetles are even able to shiver properly, rhythmically contracting their flight muscles without moving their wings, but this is not the same as shivering in homoithermous animals as these are trying to maintain a *constant* temperature, rather than to increase it.

The social insects—bees, wasps, ants and termites—have developed temperature regulation by communal action and can regulate the temperature of their nests often to within very narrow limits. Ants block the entrance of the nest with earth if the air gets too hot or too cold but honeybees block the hive door with their bodies, forming a living plug. During the summer the nest is kept at 94°–95° F. Temperature is raised above that of the surroundings by the heat given off by the bees inside the hive and if the hive gets too hot, some worker bees stand at the entrance, facing inwards and beating their wings. Hot air is drawn out and cooler air leaks in through cracks in the hive wall. If the temperature continues to rise, water is brought in and sprinkled over the top of the combs. It evaporates and cools the surrounding air which sinks, flowing past the combs. In the winter the hive temperature fluctuates in a daily cycle. As soon as the temperature drops to 56° F the bees are stimulated into activity. The hive warms to 78° F, then activity ceases and it cools again. If the outside temperature is cold for a very long time the bees may use up their stores of honey trying to keep warm and so perish.

A steady body temperature is essential to the developing offspring of many animals, especially if they are homoithermous. If a hen's egg gets cold it will never hatch as the embryo within dies. It is a matter of general knowledge that birds keep their eggs warm by incubating them, but incubation is more than just sitting on the nest. The temperature of the eggs must be controlled very carefully. Just before they are laid the parent birds lose feathers from areas on the breast called the brood patches. These patches, now bare, are plentifully supplied with blood vessels and keep the eggs warm. At intervals the eggs are turned over so that they are warmed evenly and kept near the body temperature of the incubating parent. This is a passive process, the bird does not measure the temperature of its eggs, although in bad weather it has been found that birds spend more time on their nests and are less willing to fly away if disturbed. In the tropics, on the other hand, it is sometimes necessary to keep the eggs cool and the parents stand over the nest shading the eggs from the sun. The Egyptian plover even waters its eggs. They are laid on the bare ground and buried under sand in the daytime to keep the sun off them. If the sand becomes too hot the parents fetch water from a nearby river or pool and regurgitate it over the buried eggs.

The behaviour of the Egyptian plover may be surprising but it pales beside the complicated nesting behaviour of the Australian mallee fowl which goes to incredible lengths to incubate its eggs, when there appears to be no reason why it could not incubate them in the normal way. The mallee fowl belongs to a family of birds called megapodes, literally bigfeet, and lives in the inland dry scrubland of Australia. Most megapodes bury their eggs in the ground where they are kept warm by natural heat. The junglefowl, for instance, lay their eggs in a pit which is filled in with sand. The eggs are kept warm by the sun heating the sand. In the Solomon Islands and New Britain junglefowl lay their eggs in soil which is warmed by volcanic steam and one species of junglefowl makes a mound of leaf mould in which to lay its eggs. The leaf mould rots and ferments, warming up internally like a pile of grass cuttings.

The mallee fowl goes further than this and actually controls the temperature of its nest mound. There is no leaf mould in the dry country where it lives and so it manufactures its own. The male digs a large hole, up to 15 ft in diameter and 3 ft deep, and fills it with dead leaves, twigs and so on gathered from a radius of 50 yd. After the pile has been wetted by rain it is covered with sand and left to ferment. In the spring the mallee fowl attracts females to his compost-heap and mates with them. They lay their eggs in a nest in the mound and depart leaving the male to tend the eggs for the incredibly long eleven-month incubation period. During this time the mallee fowl's life is devoted to temperature regulation.

At the beginning of the incubation period fermentation is rapid and the mound is hot, but later the process slows down so the mallee fowl has to arrange the mound to lose or conserve heat as necessary, maintaining the temperature of the eggs at around 92° F. The temperature of the sand and vegetation is tested by taking samples in the bill which contains temperature receptors. When fermentation is proceeding strongly the temperature is reduced by digging out some of the material and letting the heat escape. When the sun is very hot there is also a danger of overheating and the sand is scraped on to the mound to act as an insulating blanket. In the autumn the sun's rays are weaker and fermentation slows down so the mallee fowl digs away the sand letting the sun's heat penetrate to the eggs. Meanwhile it rakes over the scattered sand so that it warms thoroughly in the sun and can keep the eggs warm when it is pushed back into the hole at night. These are only the bare outlines of the mallee fowl's task. Until the chicks hatch and fight their way to the surface, it is constantly checking the temperature of the sand and vegetation and making the necessary adjustments to the mound.

Unlike birds and animals in previous examples, the mallee fowl is altering the environment of its offspring rather than that of its own body but, nevertheless, the temperature sense is still being used for temperature regulation and the temperature receptors have been acting as contact receptors. A few animals, however, use their temperature receptors as distance receptors to gain information about objects in their environment some way from their bodies. Blood-sucking animals such as ticks and bugs detect the warmth of their hosts' bodies. Bugs have been found to be able to detect an object at blood heat from a distance of 6 in. As a bug comes near the object, its antennae turn until they both point towards it. The bug turns so that it is pointing in the same direction as its antennae and 'follows' them towards the warm object. The bug has simple temperature receptors in its antennae and it is guided towards a warm object by taxic behaviour. Some snakes, however, have temperature receptors grouped together to form a sense organ that enables them to find out more about their environment by temperature sensing than any other animal.

The family of pit-vipers, which includes such venomous snakes as the moccasins and rattlesnakes, is so named because of the two facial pits that lie between the eyes and nostrils. Each pit is a hollow, $\frac{1}{4}$ in deep and $\frac{1}{8}$ in across at the opening, with a thin membrane stretched across the bottom. Within the membrane there are large numbers of temperature receptors, 500–1,500 packed together in 1 sq mm. Thus the facial pit is in some ways like a simple eye. The membrane containing the receptors is like a retina and the direction of a warm body can be determined since the overhanging lip of the pit casts heat 'shadows'

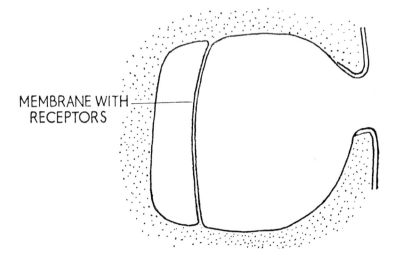

MEMBRANE WITH RECEPTORS

Fig 31   Diagram of the facial pit of a pit viper. The receptors in the membrane are sensitive to heat coming through the narrow opening. Some idea of the direction of a warm or cold object is obtained by the 'heat shadow' cast by the overhanging walls of the opening on the membrane. The field of 'view' of the two pits overlaps so that there exists the equivalent of stereoscopic vision, enabling the range to be ascertained.

The temperature receptors are extremely sensitive, responding to temperature changes of 0·002° C and allowing a snake to detect objects about 0·1° C warmer or cooler than their background. Rattlesnakes, for instance, can detect the warmth of a human hand from a distance of 1 ft. The possession of sensitive temperature organs is very useful to those animals which hunt warm-blooded prey at night. The prey is tracked by scent, but the facial pits guide the final strike.

CHAPTER ELEVEN

Electric currents and magnetic fields

The ability of fish to generate electric currents was known to the Ancient Greeks, although they did not know that the numbing shocks that fishermen received from the electric rays were caused by electricity. It was thought that the fish emitted a poisonous effluence from their veins which congealed the blood of anyone touching it. Also known to the Ancients was the electric catfish that lives in the rivers and lakes of tropical Africa. The Arab name for it is *ra'ad*, the shaker, and since the eleventh century, Arabs have used it for electrotherapy, pressing the live fish to various parts of the body as a cure for all sorts of aches and pains. The Romans made similar use of the electric rays in the treatment of gout and headaches.

Together with the electric eel of South America these fishes have organs in their bodies capable of discharging powerful electric shocks. The electric catfish can discharge up to 650 volts from electric organs which are formed from muscles. The contraction of a normal muscle starts by small charges, called action potentials, spreading over the surface of the muscle fibre like the receptor potential spreading over a receptor. In the electric organs of fishes the powers of contraction have been lost and the action potentials greatly increased. The fibres in an electric organ are not slender, like muscle fibres, but platelike and are arranged like the cells in a battery. As in a battery, the individual charges of the plates are combined to make one powerful discharge. The action potential of each plate is only about

0·1 volt, but the thousands of plates in the electric organ of an electric eel can be stimulated simultaneously to produce a large shock.

The three electric fishes, already mentioned, use their spectacular electric shock to stun their prey, but other fishes have been found to generate much weaker currents, too weak to shock their prey and often only detectable by instruments. Most, if not all, skates and rays have electric organs in their tails; the electric ray differing from the rest in producing a strong shock. Other electric fishes include the stargazers of the coasts of North America; the mormyrid fishes, such as the 'elephant-trunk' fishes of Africa; and the gymnotid fishes, which include knife-fishes, and the electric eel, of South America. The purpose of the weak currents produced by these fishes was a mystery until it was suggested that the fishes might be able to detect distortions in the electric field around their bodies and so be able to locate obstacles or prey.

The Nile fish, a strange-looking fish with a waving fin down the length of its back, has been known for over 100 years to have an electric organ. Then in 1951 Dr H. W. Lissmann of Cambridge University undertook to study their behaviour closely. Nile fish do not swim like most other fish by beating the tail, but by rippling the dorsal fin while the body is held rigid. They can glide backwards or forwards with equal ease manœuvring past obstacles without any difficulty. Their home is in muddy rivers and they hunt by night for smaller fishes. In these conditions eyesight is of little use and it would seem reasonable to suppose that Nile fish use some other sense to hunt their prey and avoid obstacles.

Dr Lissmann showed that Nile fish use their electric organs to detect objects around them and that similar mechanisms are used by other fishes with electric organs. If a pair of electrodes connected to an oscilloscope is lowered into an aquarium containing a Nile fish, electric discharges are immediately picked up. They are emitted at a steady rate of 300 per second and each one spreads out through the surrounding water forming an electric field like the field around a bar magnet, with the positive pole at the head of the fish and the negative pole at the tail. Any object in the water disturbs the electric field but it had to be shown that Nile fish were sensitive to their weak electric fields and that they used them to detect objects. They were found to react to small magnets moved about near their aquarium, and if their own discharges were recorded and played back they attacked the electrodes. Some conditioning experiments were then carried out to find out whether the Nile fish could detect objects near them. Two tubes of porous clay were put in the aquarium. One was filled with tapwater or some other conducting medium and the other was filled with a non-conductor such as wax or glass. The fish was trained to come to the conducting pot by rewarding it with a lump of meat and it soon learnt to come to the conducting pot and ignore the non-conductor. By changing the contents of the pots it was found that the Nile fish could discern the presence of a glass rod 2 mm in diameter in one of the pots. Such a fine rod can cause only a minute change in the fish's electric field, so its ability to detect it shows extremely fine sensitivity.

The sense organs used to detect the electric fields lie in the skin of the head and are very much like lateral line organs. They are minute jelly-filled pits with receptors at the bottom. The skin of Nile fish is thick and conducts electricity very badly but the jelly conducts well and so acts as an accessory organ collecting and concentrating the electric currents.

The discovery of the mechanism responsible for the Nile fishes' sensitivity to electric fields was shortly followed by that of the function of the ampullae of Lorenzini in skates and rays. In Chapter One it was mentioned that these sense organs had at one time been thought to be temperature receptors or pressure receptors, but eventually were found to be electric receptors. Like the sense organs in the head of a Nile fish they consist of a group of sense cells at the bottom of a jelly-filled tube. Similar organs have been found in other electric-sensitive fish such as the African 'elephant-trunk' fishes and the American knife fishes.

Figure 32 illustrates how non-conducting and conducting objects alter the pattern of the electric field around the head of a fish, and so, presumably, affect the pattern of nerve impulses coming from the receptors. How this pattern is used to detect the position of the object accurately, which from the proven ability of these fish to avoid obstacles we must assume to be possible, is quite unknown. The part of the brain linked to the sense organs is extremely large and must be capable of analysing the complicated data coming from the sense organs. Its job is made easier by the fish's method of locomotion. Fish usually beat their tails from side to side but most of the fishes that use electric currents keep their bodies in an almost straight line as they swim. It must be more than coincidence that this alternative way of swimming has been developed by unrelated electric

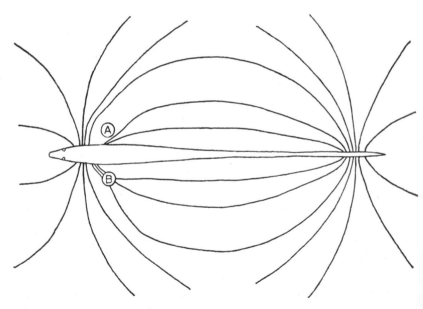

Fig 32 The electric organs in the tail of this knife fish generate a field like that around a bar magnet. The electric receptors in the head region detect distortions caused by objects near the fish. (a) is a poor conductor spreading the lines of force and (b) is a good conductor concentrating them

fishes. The electric organs of rays and skates lie in a rigid, narrow tail and they swim by flapping their pectoral fins and many of the mormyrid and gymnotid fishes, including the Nile fish and knife fishes, keep their tails straight and propel themselves by undulations in long fins on their backs or bellies. The advantage of this method of propulsion is that the electric field is not distorted as it would be if the tail was moved from side to side in swimming, and the difficulties of analysing incoming information by the brain are kept to a minimum.

A common habit of these fish is living in muddy water or being active at night. Their eyes are small so that the electric senses must be valuable, although it has yet to be shown that some species, including the skates, actually make use of their electric senses. Avoiding obstacles and finding prey may not be the only function of the electric senses. It may be found that the electric sense is used to convey signals in aggressive behaviour or courtship, as are the other senses. Nile fish, for instance, have been found to alter the frequency of their electric discharge if their original discharge is recorded and played back to them, so that it seems they can avoid jamming each other's signals.

The electric sense is very much a 'new sense'. Nearly thirty years ago it was unknown and its exploration has led to the discovery of a completely new type of sense organ. The electric sense is quite different from the other sense organs discussed in this book because they are possessed in some form by ourselves, although other animals may use them for different purposes. We may have difficulty appreciating how a bat navigates by echolocation or a bee by polarised light, but electric fishes live in an utterly alien world.

Since Dr Lissmann found that the Nile fish were sensitive to weak currents another mysterious, but perhaps related, sense has been discovered. In Chapter Seven, the comment was made that birds may possibly be able to navigate by the earth's magnetic field. There is no sound proof to show that they are sensitive to magnetic fields, but a few more primitive animals have been found to respond to weak magnetic fields. In northern

Australia the nests of certain species of termites are always built with the long axis lying north–south, so that a group of nests looks like a fleet of ships at anchor, each ship riding with its bows to the wind. A suggested reason for this orientation is that the broad sides of the nests, by facing east and west, catch the weak morning and evening sun which helps to keep the nest warm. There is no proof of this and other termite nests are known to be independent of outside temperature. The walls are very thick and the air temperature inside is regulated by the activities of the termites, in much the same way as the temperature of a bee hive is regulated.

It is, however, known that individual termites of some species are sensitive to magnetic fields. When in their nest they take up positions parallel, or in some species at right angles, to the earth's magnetic field. This might explain why the nests are orientated along the earth's field, for if the termites are facing north or south they will tend to build the nest along a north–south line. When kept in an iron box the termites lose their orientation and if a powerful magnet is placed under the floor of their cage they change position so that they lie along the new lines of force. Other animals can be led off course if a magnet is placed near them, including such diverse animals as a pond snail, a flatworm and a single-celled protozoan.

The mystery is not only why these animals orientate by magnetic fields but how they sense the magnetism. So far no sense organ or receptor has been found to respond to magnetic fields. A magnetic sense may, however, eventually be found to be quite widespread among animals, and if this is so, there is no reason to believe that it will be the last sense we shall discover. It has already been suggested that some humans are sensitive to radio waves and in 1968 it was found that the feathery antennae of some night-flying moths are sensitive to light although they have no cornea, lens or retina which are usually associated with a light-sensitive organ.

At the moment we are living in a golden age of biology. Exciting advances are being made in all fields of biological research, spurred on by the application of the latest tools from other sciences, such as electron microscopes and computers. Startling advances are being made in molecular biology, the biology of populations and social behaviour, but sense-organ physiology is also progressing rapidly. Intricate mechanisms are being revealed so it is now becoming possible to explain the behaviour of animals in terms of the capabilities and limitations of their sense organs rather than assuming that their view of the world is the same as ours. But as information accumulates more problems arise and, for all the knowledge we possess, each chapter in this book is incomplete since it has to be admitted that we do not yet know, in complete detail, how any sense organ works or even what purpose some of them serve. Eventually we will know how termites sense the earth's magnetic field and even why they respond to it, but by that time new and equally mysterious senses will no doubt have been discovered.

Bibliography

Amoore, J. E. 'Psychophysics of odor', *Cold Spring Harbour Symp Quant Biol*, 30 (1965), 623–38

Adler, J. 'Chemotaxis in *Escherischia coli*', *Cold Spring Harbour Symp Quant Biol*, 30 (1965), 289–92

Barrows, W. M. 'The reactions of an orb-weaving spider *Epeira sclopetaria* Clerck, to rhythmic vibrations of its web', *Biol Bull*, 29 (1915), 316–26

Beament, J. W. C. (ed). 'Biological receptor mechanisms', *Symposia of the Society for Experimental Biology*, No XVI (Cambridge, 1962)

Bell, G. H., Davidson, J. N., Scarborough, H. *Textbook of Physiology and Biochemistry* (Livingstone, 1961)

Belton, P. and Kempster, R. H. 'A field test on the use of sound to repel the European corn-borer', *Entomologia experimentalis et applicata*, 5 (1962), 281–8

Benzinger, T. H. 'The human thermostat', *Scientific American*, 204 (1961), 134–47

Bradshaw, S. D. and Main, A. R. 'Behavioural attitudes and regulation of temperature in *Amphibolurus* lizards', *J Zool*, 154 (1968), 193–222

Brown, F. A. 'Responses of the planarian, *Dugesia*, and the protozoan, *Paramecium*, to very weak horizontal magnetic fields', *Biol Bull*, 123 (1962), 264–81

Brown, M. E. (ed). *The physiology of fishes, Vol 2—Behaviour* (Academic Press, New York, 1957)

Bullock, T. H. and Diecke, F. P. J. 'Properties of an infra-red receptor', *J Physiol*, 134 (1956), 47–87

Bullock, T. H. and Fox, W. 'The anatomy of the infra-red sense-organ in the facial pit of pit-vipers', *Quart J Micr Sci,* 98 (1957), 219–34

Calhoun, J. B. 'Population density and social pathology', *Scientific American,* 206 (1962), 139–48

Crisp, D. J. 'Barnacles', *Science Journal,* 3 (1967), 69–73

Düecker, G. 'Colour vision in mammals', *J Bombay Nat History Soc,* 61 (1964), 572–86

Dunning, C. D. 'Warning sounds of moths', *Z für Tierpsychol,* 25 (1968), 129–38

Emlen, J. T. and Penney, R. L. 'Distance navigation in the Adélie penguin', *Ibis,* 106 (1964), 417–31

Evans, P. R. 'Reorientation of passerine night migrants after displacement by the wind', *British Birds,* Vol 61 No 7 (1968), 281–303

Ewer, R. F. *Ethology of Mammals* (Logos, 1968)

Finkelstein, D. and Grüsser, O-J. 'Frog retina: detection of movement', *Science, N.Y.,* 150 (1965), 1050–1

Flock, A. 'Transducing mechanism in the lateral line canal organ receptors', *Cold Spring Harbour Symp Quant Biol,* 30 (1965), 133–45

von Frisch, K. 'Recent advances in the study of the orientation of the honey bee', *The Bulletin of Animal Behaviour,* No 9 (1951)

Gary, N. E. 'Chemical mating attractants in the queen honey bee', *Science,* 136 (1962), 773–4

Gesteland, R. C. 'The mechanics of smell', *Discovery* (February 1966), 29–34

Griffin, D. R. *Listening in the Dark* (Yale University Press, 1958)

Griffin, D. R., Webster, F. A. and Michael, C. R. 'The echolocation of flying insects by bats', *Anim behav,* 8 (1960), 141–54

Gould, E., Nevus, N. C. and Novick, A. 'Evidence for echolocation in shrews', *J Exp Zool,* 156 (1964), 19–38

Hamburger, V. 'Versuche über Komplementär—Farben be Elbritzen (*Phoxinus laevis*)', *Zvergleich Physiol,* 4 (1926), 286–304

Haskell, P. T. *Insect Sounds* (Witherby, 1961)

Hasler, A. D. and Larsen, J. A. 'The homing salmon', *Scientific American*, 193 (1955), 72–6

Henson, O. W. 'The activity and function of the middle-ear muscles in echo-locating bats', *J Physiol*, 180 (1965), 871–87

Horridge, G. A. and Boulton, P. S. 'Prey detection by Chaetognatha via a vibration sense', *Proc Royal Soc*, Series B, 168 (1967), 413–19

Ilse, D. 'New observations on responses to colours by egg-laying butterflies', *Nature*, 140 (1937), 544

Jenkins, M. F. 'On the method by which *Stenus* and *Dianous* (Coleoptera: Staphylinidae) return to the banks of a pool', *Trans Roy Entom Soc London*, 112 (1960), 1

Kalmus, H. 'The discrimination by the nose of the dog of individual human odours and in particular of the odours of twins', *Brit J Anim Behav*, 3 (1955), 25–31

Lees, A. D. 'The sensory physiology of the sheep tick *Ixodes ricinus* L.', *J Exp Biol*, 25 (1948), 145–207

Lettvin, J. Y. and Gesteland, R. C. 'Speculation on smell', *Cold Spring Harbour Symp Quant Biol*, 30 (1965), 217–25

Levick, M. G. *Antarctic Penguins: A study of their social habits* (Heinemann, 1914)

Lissmann, H. W. 'On the function and evolution of electric organs in fish', *J Exp Biol*, 35 (1958), 156–91

Lissmann, H. W. and Machin, K. E. 'The mechanism of object location in *Gymnarchus niloticus*', *J Exp Biol*, 35 (1958), 451–86

Machin, K. E. and Lissmann, H. W. 'The mode of operation of the electric receptors in *Gymnarchus niloticus*', *J Exp Biol*, 37 (1960), 801–11

Matthews, G. V. T. *Bird Navigation* (Cambridge, 1968)

Medway, Lord. 'The function of echonavigation amongst swiftlets', *Anim Behav*, 15 (1967), 416–20

Mrosovsky, N. 'How turtles find the sea', *Science Journal* (November 1967), 53–7

Mrosovsky, N. and Shettleworth, S. J. 'Wavelength preferences and brightness cues in the water finding behaviour of sea turtles', *Behaviour*, 32 (1968), 211–57

Muntg, W. R. A. 'Microelectrode recordings from the diencephalon of the frog (*Rana pipiens*) and a blue-sensitive system', *J Neurophysiol*, 25 (1962), 699–711

Muntg, W. R. A. 'Effectiveness of different colours of light in releasing the positive phototactic behaviour of frogs, and a possible function of the retinal projection to the diencephalon', *J Neurophysiol*, 25 (1962), 712–20

Murray, R. W. 'The response of the ampullae of Lorenzini of elasmobranchs to electrical stimulation', *J Exp Biol*, 39 (1962), 119–28

Norris, K. S., Prescott, J. H., Asa-Dorian, P. V. and Perkins, P. 'An experimental demonstration of echo-location behavior in the porpoise *Tursiops truncatus* (Montagu)', *Biol Bull*, 120 (1961), 163–76

Palmer, E. and Weddell, G. 'The relation between structure, innervation and function of the skin of the bottle nose dolphin (*Tursiops truncatus*)', *Proc Zoo Soc*, 143 (1964), 553–68

Pearcy, W. G., Meyer, S. L. and Munk, O. 'A "four-eyed" fish from the deep-sea: *Bathylychnops exilis* Cohen, 1958', *Nature*, 207 (1965), 1260–1

Pumphrey, R. J. 'Hearing in insects', *Biol Rev*, 15 (1940), 107–32

Quilliam, T. A. 'The mole's sensory apparatus', *J Zool*, 149 (1966), 76–88

Ransome, R. D. 'The distribution of the greater horse-shoe bat, *Rhinolophus ferrum-equinum*, during hibernation, in relation to environmental factors', *J Zool*, 154 (1968), 77–112

Roeder, K. D. 'Behaviour of free flying moths in the presence of ultrasonic pulses', *Anim Behav*, 10 (1962), 300–4

Roeder, K. D. and Treat, A. E. 'Ultrasonic reception by the tympanic organ of noctuid moths', *J Exp Zool*, 134 (1957), 127–57

Romanes, G. J. *Mental evolution in Animals* (Keagan Paul, 1885)

Rushton, W. A. H. 'Chemical basis of colour vision and colour blindness', *Nature*, 206 (1965), 1087–91

Tansley, K. *Vision in Vertebrates* (Chapman & Hall, 1965)

Treat, A. E. 'The reaction time of noctuid moths to ultrasonic stimulation', *J New York Entom Soc*, 64 (1956), 165–71

Walcott, C. 'The effect of the web on sensitivity in the spider, *Achaeanaria tepidariorum* (Koch)', *J Exp Biol*, 40 (1963), 595–611

Walcott, C. and Van der Kloot, W. G. 'The physiology of the spider vibration receptor', *J Exp Zool*, 141 (1959), 191–244

Webster, F. A. and Griffin, D. R. 'The role of the flight membranes in insect capture by bats', *Anim Behav*, 10 (1962), 332–40

Wenzel, B. M. 'Olfactory prowess of the kiwi', *Nature*, 220 (1968), 1133–4

Wever, E. G. and Bray, C. W. 'A new method for the study of hearing in insects', *J comp cell Physiol*, 4 (1933), 79–93

Wigglesworth, V. B. *The principles of Insect Physiology* (Methuen, 1953)

Wigglesworth, V. B. and Gillett, J. D. 'The function of the antennae of *Rhodnius prolixus* and the mechanism of orientation to the host, and, Confirmatory experiments', *J Exp Biol*, 11 (1934), 120–39, 408–10

Wilson, E. O. 'Pheromones', *Scientific American*, 208 (1963), 100–14

Wolken, J. J. 'The photoreceptors of Arthropod eyes', *Symp zool soc Lond*, 23 (1968), 113–33

Wright, R. H. *The Science of Smell* (George Allen & Unwin, 1964)

Index